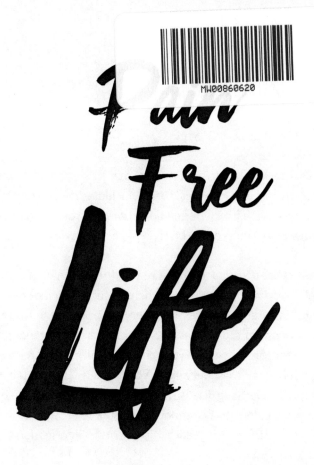

Pain Free Life

Eliminate Chronic Pain and Get Back
to a **Younger** More **Active** You!

by

TRAVIS PERRET

Pain Free Life
Eliminate chronic pain
and get back to a
younger more active you!

Con-Pan Press
7802 Foster
Overland Park, KS 66204

Cover and Interior Design: Matthew Nance, www.nanced.com

ISBN: 978-0-692-95603-8

Acknowledgements

First, I would like to thank the thousands of clients with whom I have worked over the last 20 years. The friendships I've made and the enjoyment I have gained from your successes have enlightened my life.

I would like to thank my wife. She is the voice of reason, when I am the voice of dreams. She helps to keep our family ship afloat.

Thank you to my parents, Steve and Artis Perret. They have always believed in me, even when times were hard. Without their help, I would not be where I am today. Their support in sports, school, business and life makes me who I am today. They instilled in me a mindset of working hard and never giving up. I hope to be as good a parent as they have been and are to me. To all those who have helped in making this book a reality, thank you. I have used many friends and clients as sounding boards and editors in getting this project finished.

Thank you to: Vivien Jennings, Ned and Patti Kehde, Kim and Scott Wedman, Betsy Zindle, Dr. Michelle Robin, Dr. Henry Marquardt and many others I'm sure I have forgotten to name.

Lastly, to the many other practitioners whom I have known along the way who care deeply for their clients and have given me advice or have trusted me enough to refer their clients to me: Thank you for your trust!

TABLE OF CONTENTS

1 | Chapter 1
Pain: The Red Light

15 | Chapter 2
Posture, Alignment and Function

31 | Chapter 3
Move Correctly, Feel Better

49 | Chapter 4
The Pain-Free Life Program

63 | Chapter 5
What It Takes

79 | Chapter 6
Corrective Exercises for Your Pain

FOREWARD

By Scott Wedman
Two Time NBA All-Star
Two Championships with Boston Celtics 1984 & 1986

Travis Perret's skills as a corrective exercise therapist are unparalleled. As a professional NBA basketball player for 13 years, I was exposed to the cutting edge of therapy and rehabilitation. I took pride in being one of the best-conditioned players on the team when showing up for training camp every fall. In the mid 70's through the 80's my weight lifting, yoga, visualization and focus on diet were not the norms for professional basketball players. I know that all of these were instrumental in my success in a very physical and demanding sport.

On retiring from the NBA, the demands of a normal life as a businessman and a coach presented challenges to my health that I had not anticipated. Exercising was no longer my primary focus. With a more sedentary lifestyle, sitting at a desk for hours- or sitting in a coach's chair- and then deciding to go workout at the same level I was used to brought on back problems, including a bulging disc. I resolved to avoid surgery if at all possible and was fortunate to be introduced to corrective exercise therapy, which lead me to Travis Perret. I have become a devout believer in exercise therapy over the last 25 years. I have been able to live an active life style, without surgery. I have had several instances when I was absolutely going to need surgery to repair my back, but each time Travis guided me back to full functionality and activity.

This is a therapy that puts you in control of your health. Travis is there to coach you through the aches and pains, but being consistent with the movements is up to you. You are given a menu with exercises that you can do anywhere at any time. Travis has become my postural and functional coach and enables me to keep doing the things I love to do.

Not only have I benefited from this therapy, but many of my friends and family have, as well. An older friend of mine, who is in his eighties, is an avid outdoorsman and had resigned himself to never being able to do his usual outdoor activities because of pain in his knees and hips. He had so many issues that he was confined to a wheel chair to get around. After Travis worked with him, he was able to resume his favorite pastimes with full function of his legs and hips.

My mom, 87 at the time, had become very unstable when walking because of weakness in her knees and hips, and even though she resisted, she was a candidate for using a walker. After several sessions with Travis, her stability returned, and she was able to walk without pain and without assistance.

It does not matter what your age is, you can benefit from this unique and empowering therapy!

FOREWORD

If chronic pain issues are limiting your life, I would highly recommend reading this book and doing the exercises provided. They are easy to do and a great first step toward moving better and feeling better.

INTRODUCTION

On a visit home for the holidays, I could see that my dad was having some problems. He was attempting to hide it, but I could see him wincing from pain when he tried to move. When I inquired about what was going on, he mentioned he was having severe nerve pain down the leg and intense back pain. It was so intense that he could not stand up straight without shooting pain, and putting on his socks and shoes were nearly impossible. His doctors were telling him a nerve was being pinched in his low back and he might have to have a lumbar fusion.

He has always had physically demanding jobs to provide for our family. He worked as a bricklayer early in his life, then worked in the oil fields of western Kansas, and eventually became a long haul truck driver. The high physical demands of his life had caught up with him, and his back was paying the price.

As we talked I was able to dig deeper into the cause of what was happening. His doctors were telling him because the discs in his low back had moved; constant pressure was placed on his nerve and was firing nerve pain into his back and down his leg. His doctor recommended two things: surgery and quitting his job.

I had just graduated from college and was working in San Diego, CA for the country's leading non-medical chronic pain clinic. This is where I first experienced the concept of how corrective exercises can help with chronic pain. I also learned the importance of teaching people how to take responsibility for their health and how important their personal involvement in the healing process is. I teach my clients everyday that they know their body better than anyone else and we have to listen to what it is telling us. When you are proactive and involved with the process of healing and you are willing to take the necessary steps to achieve that goal you will feel better and move better than you ever have.

I asked my dad if he would be willing to try some exercises before quitting his job and having surgery. He said, "Absolutely!" He was in so much pain he would give anything a try.

I gave him several exercises that he did every day, and within a couple of weeks he was starting to feel better. I modified the exercises a few times over the following weeks and by the next month his pain was gone and he was feeling amazingly better. He was feeling so much better and it happened so quickly we were all amazed. Even to this day he tells me that when he finishes work, he does a couple of the exercises I gave him just to make sure he continues to feel better.

Helping my dad changed my life. It gave me a more defined purpose of what I wanted to do with my life and for my career. Helping him avoid back surgery and allowing him to keep working changed the way I looked at what I was doing. It opened my eyes to the power of postural and alignment exercises. It transformed my attitude from having a job to having a passion. A passion to help guide and mentor people who have chronic pain to get back to doing what they love to do and lead a more fulfilling life without the burden and limitations of chronic pain. Teaching people that there is hope and they can feel better, move better and live better.

Since then I have dedicated over 20 years to helping people who have chronic pain regain their lives. I have studied and worked with many different types of techniques, programs, and methods throughout those 20 years. Through those experiences and studies, I have designed a process that improves posture, corrects joint and bone alignment and helps people who have had many years of chronic pain feel better than they ever have. This process can eliminate chronic pain, make you feel younger and more vibrant, and keep you active and fit throughout your whole life.

This book is not for everyone. If you believe that you are just getting old and you should just sit around and live with your pain, this book is not for you. If you believe pain pills and surgery is the only option, this book is not for you. This book is for the person who wants to be as active as they possibly can while they grow older gracefully. If you want to lead an active life and do things such as play with your kids or grandkids and not have to worry about chronic pain, you will love this book. If you are the type of person who has been active most your life and now you are limited in your movements because of experiencing chronic pain, this book is for you.

You don't have to slow down because you are experiencing chronic pain. You can be active again—or even more active than in recent years—if you are proactive and take the proper steps to achieve that goal.

In fact, being active is essential. You just have to take steps to ensure you can. Even if you don't have major chronic pain and want to insure that your body is prepared to stay active throughout your life, this book is for you.

If you are an orthopedic surgeon, physical therapist, chiropractor, personal trainer, or have a job in which you help people through physical movement, this book is for you. It is a tool you can use to help your clients feel and move better.

The goal of this book is to get you out of pain and back to doing what you love. To get you back to having an active lifestyle without physical limitations. All too often my new clients tell me they have tried everything and nothing has helped. They have been through the traditional medical route of painkillers, X-rays, MRIs and other therapies, and nothing has helped. They are at the point where they don't know what to do and feel hopeless.

You may be in this desperate situation, as well. This book has been written to give you hope…because there is a solution to fixing your chronic pain. You can feel younger, be more active, and do the things in life that make you happy, without the use of painkillers and needless surgeries.

The extraordinary transformations I have witnessed in clients who have experienced 20 or 30 years of chronic pain would amaze you. I have seen clients with such severe back pain that it limits every aspect of their daily life, from putting on their socks to brushing their teeth. They dream of being able to play golf again, of being able to get back into the garden, or of taking a walk around the block without pain. When I tell them that they are going to fix their pain AND be able to do what they love better than before, they often look at me in disbelief.

This book is not about some miracle technique or magic solution that cures chronic pain. It is about a concept that, if applied on a daily basis, will change your life. I wanted to write a book that would give people who suffer from chronic pain a tool to feel better. In eliminating chronic pain and feeling better there are no miracles. I'm going to give you a plan that could decrease your pain dramatically if you implement it through consistent effort.

As the common saying goes, every journey starts with a first step. I hope this book is your first step to feeling better.

Some knowledgeable authors warned me that trying to sell something to the readers could be the demise of a very well intended book. Well, I am selling something: I am selling the idea that there is a better way to help people who have chronic pain than what is being offered in our traditional medical paths.

Injections, joint replacements, and pain pills are not fixing the problem; they're merely masking the symptoms. These are short-term solutions to a long-term problem.

When you take responsibility for your pain and become proactive in the process of fixing it, you will transform your life. When you take steps on a consistent and persistent basis to overcome your issues, you will transform your life. When you refuse to live a life of pain and limitations, you will transform your life.

There are many pieces to the puzzle of eliminating chronic pain, such as hydration, diet, and sleep, to name a few. At Exercise Therapy of Kansas City, my clinic where we see clients, we think the most important puzzle piece is posture and alignment.

This book focuses on the physical side of chronic pain and how improving these aspects can lead you to a new life—a new life of feeling younger, being more active, and doing the things in life that make you happy - - without limitations.

While I work specifically on the physical aspects associated with muscle function and biomechanical movement, I am also a big believer in other components of healing, one being the mental side of chronic pain. We will touch briefly on a few key mental aspects, but the majority of this book is about what you can do to change the physical limitations of your body through exercise and corrective positions.

There are many books written about the mental aspect

that are remarkable, and I've worked with people who have used those techniques and have seen great success. If you are interested in digging deeper into that side of healing, I highly recommend you look into the work of John E. Sarno, MD, starting with his book, "Healing Back Pain: The Mind-Body Connection."

One part of this book where I do take the liberty of getting into the mental aspect is in examining the three common characteristics I see in clients who get better: hope, determination, and a positive attitude. These three crucial mental attitudes are critical in getting better. Getting better is not just about having someone "fix" you, it is about you doing what it takes to go through the process and obtaining your goals. With the highs and lows of pain, your mental attitude will be important.

Introduction to the Pain-Free Life Program

The Pain-Free Life Program is a whole-body exercise therapy approach that focuses on muscle education and postural alignment to stop the chronic wearing and breaking down of joints, which lead to chronic pain. The program is specifically designed for an individual client's needs according to an assessment of the client's posture, pain, and movement. We create a process of re-educating muscles to move properly in their designed range of motion, through low-demand movements and corrective positions, and thus improve the structural integrity of the body.

Its intent is to return the human body to its natural design, based on a blueprint formed over 200,000 years ago. Long before the negative effects of sitting in cars, using cell phones, and being bombarded by negative stimuli from the human race's advance in technology, we moved with efficiency and balance. You can have proper form and function back again.

Do you find it hard to believe that you can retrain your body to be what it was 200,000 years ago? The human body's biomechanical blueprint has not changed that much in the last 200,000 years, and even less has changed in the last 10,000 years. What has changed and is changing every year is technology. As technology changes, it creates an environment of convenience and ease of use in everything we do. People no longer move as much as they are designed to move, because they don't have to. This lack of movement affects specific muscles. Muscles affect our joints. Due to technology, we no longer have to hunt and gather in order to survive.

We need to apply specifically designed movements and positions that focus on the muscles and areas that are starving for attention. We don't have to climb a tree to feel better, but we do have to stimulate the proper muscles. This can be done through low-demand, easy exercises and postural positions in the comfort of your own home.

INTRODUCTION

How to Benefit from this Book?

The exercises in the back of this book are general corrective exercise positions and movements that will start you on your journey of becoming pain-free. Every person is different, and setting a specific protocol of exercises to help chronic pain without an individual assessment is a slippery slope. An exercise that helps one person might not help another.

So we recommend that you pay close attention to your body. Listen to what your body tells you. You know your body better than anyone else. If you are doing something that hurts, stop doing it. Do not force your body to do something it does not want to do. That can only lead to other issues. If you are having problems performing the exercises in this book, I would recommend giving us a call. We can design a program that is more specific to your issues.

In the first part of the book, we will discuss concepts and ideas on why you have pain and the underlying causes of your pain. We will talk about terms such as symptoms, dysfunctions, and compensations.

The second part of the book is the exercises. This is where you have to take an active part in the process. In order to transform your life, you have to make the journey; no one else is going to make it for you. So each day you need to take that step toward feeling better.

CHAPTER 1
Pain: The Red Light

According to a study from the Institute of Medicine, 100 million Americans have pain. Chances are, if you are reading this book, you are having some type of pain. Chronic pain is an epidemic in our society. It does not get the attention cancer, heart disease, and breast cancer get because, even though chronic pain can make your life miserable, it does not kill you.

Or, I should say, directly kill you. There are many documented instances where people who have elected to get back surgery or knee surgery have died due to a complication of the surgery. Technically, the pain didn't kill them, but a major and scary side effect of surgery is death, no matter how routine or minor the surgery. We have all heard stories of an infection or a bad reaction to a medication creating complications.

Also, according to that same study from the Institute of Medicine, chronic pain affects more Americans than diabetes, heart disease, and cancer combined. Pain affects 20% of all adult Americans' sleep a few times a week or more; that is basically 42 million people who are having issues not sleeping due to pain.

The effect of chronic pain in our lives is getting out of hand, and there doesn't seem to be any traditional medical cure coming any time soon. The cure happens when we take responsibility to fix ourselves and to find our own answers. It happens when we decide to stop procrastinating and to take time out of our busy day in order to find the solution to our chronic pain. When we take the time now to focus on ourselves and not wait until it is too late.

Pain is a message to your brain that something is wrong and needs to be fixed. Like the red warning light on your car's dashboard, pain is the warning light of the body. If you don't take your car to a mechanic quickly, there could be dire consequences that could cost you dearly in the long run. Ignoring your pain signal and fighting through the pain could cause more and more problems. The sooner you address the problem, the faster you feel better and the quicker you can get to being active again.

When you get those aches and pains, your body is trying to communicate with you, trying to tell you something. Most of us have gone through our lives trying to ignore those signals, hoping they will just go away. But as you grow older, you have to be smarter about your body and listen to what it says.

Case Study: Runner with Pain

A client in his early 50s who loved to run came into my clinic. He said his early morning run got him mentally prepared for his day. He ran before the roads were cluttered with traffic, before the weather turned hot, and before all the stresses of his job kicked in. He could almost predict how his day would unfold by the way his morning run went.

Normally, he could run five or six miles without any problems, but then the pain would appear. It plagued his right hip within the first couple of miles, forcing him to stop. Yet it never hurt when he was walking or moving around during the day. He was concerned that he was creating a bigger problem by being physically active and feared he would have to stop running altogether before causing major damage.

In my office, I had him stand in front of me. Right away I could see that his right knee was pointing slightly in, while his left knee was facing slightly out. The difference in femur positions was barely noticeable but gave me a clue that there was something going on with the muscles in his hips. The hip muscles move the femur, which moves the knee.

As I did a gait analysis on him, I could see he would load his weight onto the right hip more than the left. His upper body was slightly tilted to the right when he was putting his right heel on the ground to initiate heel strike. The disparity was causing him to use one side of his body more than the other. At this point it was an issue only when he was putting the demand of running into the equation.

He was not conscious of the difference, but once I pointed it out to him, he could feel it happening with each step.

"Your fears were correct," I told him. "Ignoring this problem and continuing to run could have led to bigger issues—even to the point of needing to have your hip replaced."

His hip joints were not causing pain. The way his muscles were moving the hips, which created excessive demand on one side, was the source of the pain. The lack of proper function in certain muscles caused the hip to be limited in its ability to move properly, which caused overuse and then pain. The Pain-Free Life Program I put together targeted the muscles that engage the hips, thus stabilizing the pelvis in order to create balance on the right and left side. He did his routine every day, and in two weeks he was back to his normal runs, pain-free.

Can't I Just Take Medication?

The typical way of dealing with persistent pain is to take medications. Unfortunately, pain medications are maskers, not fixers. Some medications can decrease inflammation, but they do not work on what caused the inflammation in the first place. They do not address the source of the problem; they are just stopping the pain signal from reaching the brain. The problem is still there, but chemicals in the medications are masking it.

Sticking with the same analogy of the car's warning light, the light goes away if you cut the wire that triggers it. However, the problem that made the light turn on is still there, whether the oil is low or the engine is overheating. This concept could apply to pain medications, as well. They are cutting the signal of pain to the brain; they are not fixing the problem.

Another great example is headaches. So many things can cause headaches, and there are many different types and forms of headaches. Are you dehydrated, stressed, or are there larger issues creating the headaches? In most cases, you can take some medication to help you feel better. Many people stop there because the headache is gone. But what if you figure out why you have the headache and work at fixing the problem causing the pain and not just focus on the symptom of the head hurting? The same goes if you are using pain medications for chronic pain. You have chronic back pain and take medication for it, but to fix the source of the problem, you need to figure out why your back hurts.

One of the major reasons people come to my clinic for pain relief is the mounting problem caused by the negative side effects of their medications. The medications might be providing some relief from the pain signal, but it is only temporary. To keep getting that relief, you have to take more and more medications. That path leads to bigger issues, including damage to your liver and other vital organs.

Opioids, or prescription painkillers, use is one of the biggest epidemics in our society. It is at an all time high. According to the Department of Health & Human Services, in 2014 240 million prescriptions were written for prescription opioids. Also, according to the same information, 78 people a day die from an opioid-related overdose.

There are a lot of great medications that have saved many

lives. There are medications that have prevented and cured diseases. But painkillers are not a solution and can actually be causing more harm. When it comes to chronic pain, you have to figure out what is causing the problem and not just cover up the symptoms.

Get Back to an Active Lifestyle without Pain

Scientific studies tell us that staying active as we get older is good for us. Likewise, common sense tells us this same message. But what if you can't be active because every time you try to move you have pain?

I believe activity itself does not create pain; the way your body moves during that activity creates the pain. This means you don't have to stop the activity to make the pain go away. Instead, you can change the way your body moves during that activity in order to feel better. In other words, change the way you move so you can keep doing what you love to do. Disc herniation, bulging discs, stenosis, arthritis, bone-on-bone joints, and sciatica are a few examples of this type of chronic pain.

EXAMPLE: KNEE PAIN WHEN WALKING

Your knee starts to hurt when you walk, but you haven't injured it. This pain when walking is something that has gradually worsened over time. The pain level could have been pretty low when you first noticed it, but over the years the pain level or the frequency has been increasing.

This is happening because of improper mechanics of the knee when you are walking. The walking is not what is causing your knee to hurt, but the mechanics of your knee when walking creates the pain.

Acute Pain vs. Chronic Pain

There are basically two types of pain: acute pain and chronic pain. The general medical definition of acute pain is pain that lasts less than 30 days. The definition of chronic pain is pain that last six months or longer. But there is some gray area in distinguishing between acute and chronic pain, as well as the relationship between them.

Time really complicates pain and often makes pinpointing the cause difficult. Many times chronic pain happens years after an accident or injury. First, acute pain may erupt, and then months or years after the initial injuries heal, chronic pain appears. Often the root cause is unknown or has long been forgotten, but the effects on the body have continued to grow.

EXAMPLE: WALKING UP STAIRS

One day you are walking up some stairs, and your knee starts to hurt. This knee pain is new to you, but it would still be considered chronic pain because the source of it took years of improper knee mechanics to get to the point that taking a step one day hurt.

Often when knees hurt, people go get an X-ray, and the doctor tells them their knee joints are bone-on-bone, with no cartilage left in the knee. Wearing cartilage to this point happens over many years. Yet the pain might have only started recently.

An example of acute pain lasting longer than 30 days is when a person tears their ACL. He will have a lot of acute knee pain right away. If he elects not to have surgery to repair the ACL, the pain will subside over time. Then six months later he decides to go for a run because the pain is better, but quickly it starts to return.

Because of the injured ACL, the knee will start to hurt.

This is still labeled acute pain, even though the pain has lasted longer than 30 days. There is an injury that has not been addressed, so the problem is still there.

Other examples of acute pain that can last longer than 30 days are bone chips, torn muscles (such as rotator cuff muscles), and sprained joints.

Sometimes the results of wear on the body take years to develop, but one day you do something that sets something off. The old saying, "the straw that broke the camel's back," applies to this concept. Intense pain can erupt suddenly, caused by years of repetitive motion.

If you have a job where you have to sit for long hours and have worked in that job for many years, your hip muscles and hamstrings can tighten. When these muscles tighten, the function of the hips is limited. Bending over to pick up a pencil puts stress on the back, because the pelvis is not moving to help with the motion due to the tightness in the muscles. That is when your back goes out; or in other words, that is when the disc between the vertebrae slips and puts pressure on the nerve and creates pain.

Years of sitting tighten the muscles to the point that they lose function and become too tight to move within their designed range. When your body is confronted with a challenging task, such as bending over and picking something up, a ligament or tendon tears or a disc slips, and the pain erupts. Sitting for many years affects how your muscles function, which limits your body's ability to move properly. Picking up a pencil and having your back go out is an extreme case, but I hear it all the time. It could be bending over to pick up a grandchild or picking up the hose in the garden. A movement that is simple that you know shouldn't be causing pain.

Acute pain can force the body to focus the demand of movement to other areas to help decrease stress on the injured area. This is called compensation. Once the pain of the injury goes away, the lack of proper movement from the compensation is still present because of muscle memory. Without re-educating the muscles, the body is not able to move properly, structurally or symmetrically. Even a slight compensation performed over many years can create damage.

Life of Pain

Excessive wearing of joints over many years of misuse generally causes chronic physical pain. Let's figure out how this applies to the lives of people with chronic pain.

EXAMPLE: BACK GOES OUT

Often when your "back goes out," the story goes like this: you are in your office and drop a pencil on the floor. When you bend over to pick it up, your back "goes out." Your pain does not get better with rest and seems to get worse as time goes on.

The pencil did not hurt your back, but the way your body was bending caused stress on the discs and vertebrae.

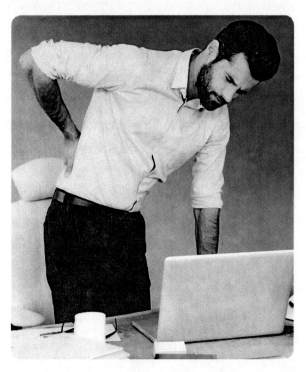

The History of a Car Accident

I often see clients who were in car accident several years before coming in to see me. The direct effects of the accident are gone; the client's broken bones, sore muscles, and other wounds have healed, or so it seems. When these clients come into my clinic, they are often complaining that they are afflicted with some kind of chronic pain, but they are not associating it to what happened in the past. They are assuming they have healed from those issues and that they no longer have effects from them.

When I do a gait analysis, I see that their hips are not working like they should. One hip could be rotating backwards much more than the other. This tells me that they are not getting the proper extension in their hip when the leg and foot are moving under them and eventually behind them.

As this unilateral hip rotation is happening, it is causing the low back to twist slightly with every step as unconscious compensation for movement limitations in the hip. This low back rotation is happening with every step they take and have been taking since starting the recovery from the accident.

When I explain this, I use the example of headlights. Let's say you have headlights on your hips. When you are moving properly, those headlights pretty much point straight ahead.

Imagine what the headlights are doing when your hips are rotating. They are pointing off in one direction with each step, causing your back to twist. The twist causes stress on the vertebrae and discs, which slowly wears them down. This twist causes muscles to become overly tight, to the point that they start to hurt on a regular basis.

The brain is smart enough to subconsciously know that your eyes are supposed to point straight ahead and look forward. In this scenario, your brain is also forcing your upper body to stay straight, so you don't fall over, while your hips and low back are twisting. The twist of the low back and the straightness of the upper body create a spot in the low back that is wearing and breaking down. This is the pivot point. The back is not causing the pain, but the way the hips are moving is causing the back to hurt.

So even after that specific injury healed, the body was never fixed of its compensation. That compensation has created chronic pain years later.

The Downward Spiral

Health for most Americans runs in cycles. Having chronic pain prevents you from moving the way you are designed to move and causes your health cycle to deteriorate. When movement causes you pain, you stop moving as much. Decrease in movement leads to even more decreased movement. Often this leads to becoming less healthy overall, and your eating habits usually become unhealthier, as well. One thing leads to the next, and you find yourself 50 or 100 pounds overweight, all because you have chronic pain. The process is like a runaway train.

CHAPTER 2
Posture, Alignment and Function

These days posture has become an overused word in the world of therapy and fitness. When I first started working with clients who had chronic pain, very few therapies were talking about how posture and function could help. They were focused on symptoms and not on the overall problem that was creating the symptom.

In understanding how posture, alignment and function can fix your chronic pain, we need to understand what they mean. We also need to understand what they tell us and how they relate to helping us determine what is happening to your body. According to the Merriam-Webster Dictionary:

Posture: the position or bearing of the body whether characteristic or assumed for a special purpose.

Posture is how we hold our body during a static position, such as sitting or standing. It is an overall view of what our body is doing. Often we state whether we have good posture or bad posture. It is a snap shot of our general positioning.

Alignment: the proper positioning or state of adjustment of parts (as of a mechanical or electronic device) in relation to each other.

Alignment is the specific details of how the joints and bones make up your posture. It looks at how each joint and bone is positioned in relation to each other.

Function: the special purpose or activity for which a thing exists or is used.

Function is how your posture and alignment allow you to move. That movement is achieved through muscles. Your muscles make your bones move. Proper function is how your body was designed to move. When your overall posture is off because of specific alignment issues, then the amount of function that happens is limited. Limitations create compensation and imbalance, which lead to chronic pain.

The key to feeling better is moving better. Chronic pain happens when we are not moving as we are designed to move. We can determine the limitations of our movement and how to fix those limitations by analyzing our overall posture and then focusing on specific issues with the alignment of our joints and bones. All that information helps us determine how our body is functioning when moving from point A to point B, or how we are moving correctly or incorrectly when swinging a golf club or taking a walk or whatever activity we like to do.

When you are sitting at a desk, you should not have to think about your shoulder position or your hip position. You should be able to sit, walk or run the way you were meant to without being concerned about how it is happening.

TRY THIS:

Stand in front of a full-length mirror. Wear a pair of shorts so you can see your kneecaps. Close your eyes and walk in place for a count of 10. Let your feet and legs move how they want.

Open your eyes and take a look at your knees and feet. If your kneecaps had eyes, where would they be looking? Are your feet straight or pointed out? Is one foot pointed out more than the other?

If they are not pointed straight ahead, this is a sign that your posture, alignment and function are limited.

Good Posture Is Natural Design

I compare posture to blinking. You don't think about blinking, it just happens. You can make yourself blink when you need to, but it should happen naturally. Posture is the same way. You can make yourself have good posture, but it should happen naturally.

Many therapies say you should concentrate on having good posture when you are sitting or when you are walking. What if your muscles don't know how to function properly in order to move your body into the proper posture? What if, after years of misinformation, they are too tight or weak to create that movement you are trying to force them to achieve?

After 10 years of sitting in an office job, one day you realize you are slouching in your chair, and you decide to sit up straight. We have all tried it. Usually this lasts for about 10 seconds, and you forget about it and go back to your normal slouching position.

But let's say you are really determined to fix your slouching. So you force sitting up to happen over and over again. You even take the next step and buy an expensive chair that is going to change the way you sit. That chair is forcing you to do something your body can't do. You force it to the point that it actually starts to hurt instead of feel good, even though sitting straight is supposed to be good for you.

Through years of unintentional training, you have educated your muscles to do the wrong thing. Sitting doesn't sound much like a workout, but it is because it is sending a signal, a stimulus to the muscles. When you are at your desk you are creating consistent bad stimuli to the muscles. Our bodies can handle bad stimuli for a short period of time, but when it happens over years and years, it creates muscle issues. Some muscles become tight, and others become weak.

Trying to convince your body to obtain better posture through force is not the answer. But what if we train your body to sit better, instead of forcing it to sit better? What if we teach the proper muscles to do the work so it happens naturally?

What if we educate the muscles that are designed to make you sit straight? This can't be done by just being aware of your posture and then forcing it to change. You have to teach your body by re-educating the muscles to do what they are designed to do.

So we have established that good posture should feel natural and happen without thinking, but what does it actually look like? Remember: posture is an overall view of what alignment is. Good posture is good alignment. Good alignment creates proper function.

Remember that old song from grade school? Your knee bone is connected to your thighbone. Your thighbone is connected to your hipbone, and so forth. I'm a big fan of that song, because it explains very simply how the whole body works together.

Viewing the body from an engineering perspective, good alignment is when the load-bearing joints of the body line up. Just like a skyscraper, the entire load-bearing structure needs to line up in order to not fall over.

How the body moves relates more to the field of engineering than to the world of science. One important term that comes from engineering and has been related to the human body is "kinetic chain." A kinetic chain is when rigid non-moving parts are put together via joints to create movement. Posture relates to the kinetic chain because everything has to be lined up and efficient to move.

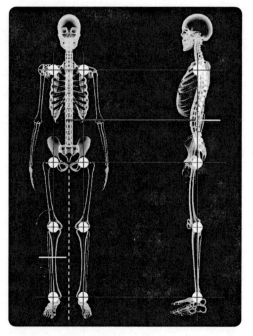

Looking at the body from the front, the ankles, knees, hips, and shoulder joints should all line up, bottom to top. We should be able to draw a line straight through all those joints, and that line should be straight on our right side and our left side. The feet should be straight—not the big toe, but the outside of our feet should be a straight line.

From the side view, the load-bearing joints should all be stacked directly on top of one another. The ankle, knee, hip, shoulder, and ear should all line up. We should have a curve in the low back, with our hips slightly tilted forward and our butt out.

This is the natural design of the human body. This is what the human body has looked like for hundreds of thousands of years. It is the position of an athletic body that is ready to move. It is the hunter and gatherer body that has allowed humans to survive for as long as we have.

Have you ever traveled to a country with less technology than in the United States, where the majority of the people still work outside? Did you take a close look at their posture? See how their shoulders are pulled back and their feet are pointed straight ahead. Their butt muscles are strong, and they have a powerful natural curve in their low back.

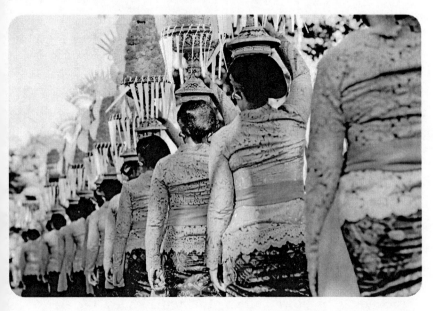

Notice how good their posture and alignment are: Look at their good shoulder position. Pay attention to their knee position and how straight their feet are as they walk. Their bodies are better aligned because their day is filled with activity and movement in order to survive and provide for their families.

Another great example that proves we are designed with good posture is looking at an infant who is just learning to walk. When my daughter was 21 months old, she started to walk consistently. As she walked, she had her shoulders back and her butt sticking out. Her belly was extended out, and her feet were always pointed straight ahead. I didn't teach her this; she just did it as she learned to walk.

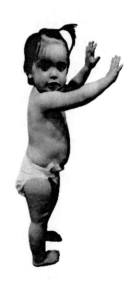

As her muscles developed from crawling and standing, she naturally progressed into good posture. We start out with good posture and good alignment, but as we grow into young adults and then mature adults, our environment changes, which changes our alignment for the worse.

When Did Good Posture Go Bad?

Technology is slowly hurting the human body. We are sitting more overall, and an hour of gym time three or four days a week is not what is needed to improve the situation if you are having chronic pain. Working out is great for the heart and lungs, but we are focused on getting you out of pain.

The blueprint of the human body is correct. When you have chronic pain, your body has deviated from that blueprint. The deviation has come from improper use of the muscles. We are not designed to sit at a computer or drive a car. We can do those movements because the body has the ability to move, but we are not meant to be in those positions for long periods of time. The body is designed to move. It is designed for climbing a tree to get to an apple or to walk several miles to get to a watering hole. Consistent changing of movements and different stimuli are what help the body feel good. When early humans hunted and gathered, they were consistently using different muscles.

I'm not suggesting you quit your job and begin providing for your family by hunting and gathering. You would probably have less chronic pain, but becoming a hunter and gatherer would be almost impossible in our day and age.

What I am advocating is that you add something to your life that counters the bad stimuli. You have to create a bridge from the hunter-gatherer posture to modern-society posture. Gym workouts and treadmills are not enough. You have to specifically target the muscles that create better alignment. When you target the postural muscles first and then go into the workout, you have created a postural bridge.

POSTURAL BRIDGE

Doing exercises that focus on restoring good posture, muscle balance, and joint alignment before your activity. This way your body performs that activity better, and the activity is better for you.

Technology Takes its Toll

The average human head weighs between 10 and 12 pounds—basically the size of a bowling ball. Think about the stress this puts on your neck when you are looking down at your phone.

A study by Kenneth K. Hansraj, chief of Spine Surgery at New York Spine Surgery and Rehabilitation Medicine in New York City, says that varying degrees of your head being forward of your shoulders increase the actual overall weight of your head. For instance, moving your head 30 degrees in front of your shoulders increases the weight of your head to 40 pounds.

According to an article published in the Daily Mail, the average person spends eight hours and 41 minutes on electronic devices a day. Looking at your phone or using a computer at your desk causes your head and neck to move forward of your shoulders. Whether you have a standing desk or a sitting desk, viewing the computer screen is affecting your head and neck.

Since this study focuses on the use of electronic devices, you might think it focuses primarily on the younger population; you

---

[1]KENNETH K. HANSRAJ, MD
CHIEF OF SPINE SURGERY
NE W YORK SPINE SURGERY & REHABILI TATION MEDICINE NEW YORK, NEW YORK
https://cbsminnesota.files.wordpress.com/2014/11/spine-study.pdf
http://www.digitaltrends.com/mobile/informate-report-social-media-smartphone-use/
http://www.pewinternet.org/2010/09/02/cell-phones-and-american-adults/

would be wrong. More and more older adults are using cell phones. In fact, a study by Pew Research Center found that 82 percent of adults between the ages of 50 and 64 own a cell phone, and 57 percent of adults age 65 and older own one.

Thus, millions of folks of all ages are using smart phones and habitually checking their email and social media accounts. All of this adds up to a recipe for head and neck pain.

Head Forward Experiment

How do you know how far your head is forward of your shoulders? Stand against a wall. If the back of your head touches the wall when your heels, butt and shoulders are on the wall, then your head is aligned properly. If the back of your head is not touching the wall, then you have a forward head position.

The key is to figure out how your body is different than the blueprint. When you have rounded shoulders, you usually know you have bad posture. Rounded shoulders are easy to see in the mirror. People who have bad posture usually know they have bad posture. It is more difficult to see when other areas are out of alignment.

That is why, in the clinic, we take a picture of all of our clients' posture. The picture allows you to see, from an outside perspective, what we are seeing from a posture point of view. We take the picture behind a plumb line which hangs from the ceiling to give us a gauge of proper alignment. Then we take additional pictures throughout the program to see how posture and alignment have improved.

All too often, our clients are surprised by what they see in the first pictures. Those who think they have good posture often don't look at how their hips or knees are aligned. They are focused on their shoulders and trying not to slouch. You have to look at every aspect and figure out how it is related to alignment and then ascertain what that says about function. For many, their posture has changed slowly over the years, and they just don't realize how bad it has become.

To Tuck or Not To Tuck

Frequently, I hear from new clients that they have been told to suck in their belly and tuck their hips to improve their posture. They try to apply this to everyday living, like when they are in the grocery store, sucking and tucking because they have been told it strengthens the abs and supports the back.

This is incorrect—sucking in your abs and tucking your hips actually can create back pain. It misaligns the hips and back, thus creating more instability over time. When the hips are tucked too far and the low back is trying to flatten, this will encourage the shoulders and head to round forward. The abs are used for some support of the back, but your back muscles support your back. Having strong abs is good, but not at the expense of your back's health. There needs to be symmetry between the front and back muscles in order to support the back. Relax and let the natural position of your abs and back do the work.

Many clients have come into our clinic with their stomach and hips tucked, and we put them in a corrective exercise position that forces them to extend their stomach and arch their back. When they stand up, their pain is gone; sometimes the solution can be as simple as that. Other times we have to combat years of training to get the muscles to change.

The evidence that proves that the suck and tuck is not natural to humans can be found in the history of the human body. Ten thousand years ago the human body wasn't sucking and tucking. We were not trying to look good; we were just trying to survive. The body is not designed to contract those muscles on a constant basis. Those muscles are meant to contract when our body needs them to perform a task.

Usually your upper back starts to tighten because of overuse, and your butt and external hip rotators tighten, decreasing hip extension; over a long period of time, this causes wearing of the hip and low back.

We also need to mention that you can have too much arch in your low back. Having too much extension in the spine can also create pain. This is usually seen in high-level athletes or people who have worked out over many years at a high level. Their hip flexors and psoas muscles have become excessively tight, causing the hips to tilt too far forward creating a big arch in the low back. The low back muscles are tight and can create compression on the lower discs.

We are all different. Our lives are different, and the histories of our bodies are different. Creating balance according to the individual needs of that specific person is important. The faster you want to feel better, the more specific the exercises need to be for your specific issues.

The Connection

Another example of bad posture negatively affecting the body is with shoulder position, rotator cuff muscle strains, or tears through chronic misuse.

Round your shoulders forward and notice how that changes your back position. Now raise one shoulder higher than the other. Basically, shrug one shoulder. Can you feel how that affects the muscles all the way down your back?

You might be forcing those changes to happen right now, but if you are experiencing back pain, incorrect shoulder positions are likely happening all the time without you realizing it.

Now stand up and roll your shoulders forward. Then raise your arms over your head. Can you feel the strain and the pressure this puts on your shoulders? If you hold your arms up for a length of time with your shoulders rounded, you can feel the muscles starting to fatigue.

BICEPS CONTRACTION EXAMPLE

Imagine if you were to bend your arm, squeeze your bicep, and hold the contraction all day. Eventually, this would start to hurt. As the pain from holding the muscle squeezed all day got worse, other areas would start to compensate to help with the contraction. Your shoulder muscles would start to burn, and your wrist and forearm would start to, as well.

If you are unable to extend your arm because you have been told to squeeze it, you would not be able turn the doorknob to open a door or reach up to get a glass of water. To perform those movements, you would have to compensate and use muscles that were not designed to perform those actions in order to accomplish that task.

Or you would have to use the other arm. Over a period of time using the other arm all the time would start to create overuse issues in that arm.

The bicep contraction example sounds silly, but it is exactly what is happening when you contract your abs and tuck your hips. That action is limiting the range of motion in your hips and vertebrae, forcing other muscles that are not designed for that kind of use to be involved.

Because of improper joint alignment of the shoulders from dysfunctional muscles (remember: muscles move bones), there is too much strain on the small muscles of the shoulder capsule. The muscles are actually fighting each other. The smaller, weaker muscles lose the battle to the bigger stronger muscles. When they lose the battle, you pull or tear a rotator cuff muscle.

Now do the opposite of that shoulder experiment, and pull your shoulders back and pin your shoulder blades together. Lift your hands over your head.

If you don't already have muscle problems like a torn rotator cuff, then you can feel how much easier it is. There is no strain and no effort to lift your arms. It feels natural and easy, just like lifting your hands over your head should feel.

That is what good posture and alignment does. It allows you to move with freedom, without stress on the muscles, and without pressure on the joints. It is a natural way to move, ingrained through thousands of years of education in our DNA.

CHAPTER 3
Move Correctly, Feel Better

Sarah came into the clinic with a herniated disc and was being told by her doctors that the only option to fix her pain was surgery. She had a close friend who had a failed back surgery and was feeling worse than before the procedure. Her friend recommended she never get the back surgery. Sarah was looking for a better option to get her life back and feel better. She had seen, from her friend, what a failed surgery could do and was willing to avoid going under the knife at all cost. On that first visit she said she was having a good day, which meant that her pain level was an **eight** on a scale of one to 10—and a 10 equaled extremely intense pain.

"What does the pain limit you from doing that you miss the most?" I asked her.

"Gardening," she answered almost immediately. "I haven't been able to tend to my flowers since I've had this pain." She put her hand on her back with a wince. "I can't bend over, and long periods of bending over send me into a back spasm."

"Well," I said, "let's see what we can do to get you back into your garden."

I had her walk around the office so that I could observe how she moved. I then had her walk with her hands on her head.

She looked a little surprised by my request, but raised her hands behind her head and walked back and forth. "What did that do to your pain level?" I asked. Her eyes lit up as she said her pain level decreased from an eight to a two.

Why and how did her pain decrease so dramatically? The answer is better alignment, which allowed better function. Better function decreased pressure on the area of pain.

By placing her hands on her head, she had changed her whole body alignment. Changing the alignment of her shoulders changed the alignment of her back, which took the pressure off the disc, giving her some much-needed relief. So much so, she didn't want to put her arms back down.

I told her that by doing a few exercises she would be able to achieve the same feeling while keeping her hands at her side. After three visits to my clinic, she was able to get back into the garden and do what she loved to do for as long as she wanted without pain. She was amazed that even though she had had years of dealing with back issues it took only three visits to see a dramatic improvement. Sometimes when the body starts working better the pain will stop instantly.

These are the same results I hope to help you achieve through the Pain-Free Life Program—results that allow you to get back to doing what you love to do and allow you to enjoy your life without a black cloud over your head.

Symmetry

GOOD ALIGNMENT IS HAVING GOOD MUSCLE SYMMETRY.

Your body's movement anatomy is naturally symmetrical. We are bipeds, meaning we have two legs that allow us to walk and run. We have two arms, two hands, and two eyes. Our right side muscles and left side muscles are a mirror of each other. The more symmetrical one side is to the other, the better we move and feel.

One of the many symptoms I hear from clients is that they are having issues with balance. They feel like they are going to fall when they walk or when they make a quick turn. That feeling of instability can make you feel old. It can also be dangerous. If you become too unstable, you can fall and break a hip or arm.

A few years ago, a client named Betty had a hip replaced, and ever since, she had been unable to walk without a significant limp. Even after her physical therapy sessions ran out and she worked with a personal trainer, she still had issues. Her hip felt fine, but her limp worsened to the point that she had to use a cane to prevent from falling.

Her biggest fear was losing her balance, falling, and breaking something. She knew friends who had fallen and never recovered; they had to spend the rest of their lives in a nursing home. She did not want that to happen to her.

After only a few sessions that focused on getting both hips

to move better, her imbalanced muscles started to function better, which led to her hips being more symmetrical. This decreased the pressure on the injured hip, and the exercises taught her other hip to work better, allowing her to walk better. She quickly forgot her cane and was starting to walk every day for exercise— something she never thought she would be able to do again. She was walking so much better, her family and friends commented on how active she had become and how much better she looked.

When we dig into the specifics of alignment, we have to look at the overall symmetry—how each side is positioned compared to the other side. Having one side different than the other causes excessive wearing and overwork; this causes inflammation, which can lead to chronic pain. When you limit your function due to not being properly symmetrical, you create an environment conducive to chronic pain.

The Hip Example

There are about 17 muscles that move the hip, with a few more that assist. All of these muscles should be symmetrical in strength, flexibility, and range of motion. Having even one or two muscles out of symmetry can cause a disparity of the pelvis.

What happens if there is a hip disparity? Each area affects the other with muscles overlapping, creating the kinetic chain. Again, like our favorite old song, the knee bone is connected to the thighbone. The thighbone is connected to the hipbone.

The hipbone is connected to the spine, and on up the line connections happen. If there is a hip disparity, this can cause the spine to be out of position. A spine out of position can cause wearing on the discs or pinching of the nerves.

Returning to our engineering analogy, imagine the Empire State Building. What if one side of the foundation of the Empire State Building was higher than the other? The whole building would tilt. People would be running around afraid that it might soon collapse.

This is what happens when you have a hip disparity. It improperly tilts the spine. The human body has an amazing ability to subconsciously try to fix any tilting. Through proprioceptors in your body, your shoulders and head will counter tilt to fix the feeling that you are about to fall. This happens on such a small scale that you might not even know you do it until years later. Years of being improperly aligned gradually build; you don't realize it has happened until one day there is too much strain on the body, and you begin to hurt.

Compensation

Compensation is a coping mechanism that we use in time of distress. We do it mentally and physically. It is what our body does to help get us through a stressful time or event until we are in a better place. Every day I see clients whose bodies have learned to cope with lack of function through compensation.

TRY THIS: WALKING EXPERIMENT

Find a hallway. Walk up and down the hallway without shoes. Take note of where you feel your feet contacting the floor. Do you feel the outside of your feet contacting the floor, or more so your heels or toes? Is the right foot different from the left foot?

Then put your hands behind your head and pull your elbows and shoulders back. What changes in how your feet contact the floor? What changes in your symptoms?

Putting your hands behind your head will change your posture by engaging the muscles down your spine and into your hips, thus changing the mechanics of your walking.

Compensation happens automatically and subconsciously, and sometimes we are aware when it happens, while at other times we have no idea that it is occurring.

An obvious example of physical compensation is when you have an injury - a sprained ankle, for instance. You limp. Your body wants to get you from point A to point B, so it does what it has to in order to get there. Other areas of the body put in extra work to compensate for the injured ankle in order to get your body to move. This can happen with shoulder, back, or knee injuries.

When clients come in for evaluations, I often dig into their physical histories. I learn what their bodies have been through to lead up to the point of chronic pain. As I evaluate their walking, I point out ways their bodies are moving improperly. They often start to connect the dots on how an old injury could be the cause. The injury may no longer be hurting, but the compensation that originally occurred has never been addressed. Years later, chronic wearing and breaking down of the compensation area creates pain.

In another example, the source of pain is not so obvious. It could be from years of lack of movement. It could be from sitting at a job all day for many years, or having a job where you are on your feet for many hours of the day. Basically, chronic pain can happen because of everyday life.

The human body and brain are amazing and instinctively smart. With a blueprint more than 200,000 years old, the human body has become so smart over those thousands of years that the medical field doesn't even understand certain ways it works. The human mind and body are like no other animal on the planet, and the way humans move is unique and deliberate. We have developed to operate very efficiently in making subconscious and conscious movement happen.

For example, let's compare our body to a turtle. The human body does not have a protective shield to hide behind until danger passes. Because we can't retreat into a hard outer shell when being attacked, the human species has had to either run from danger or stop and fight to survive. If we chose not to run or fight, we would die. Fight or flight is entrenched in our DNA. Without the ability to move, the human species would not exist.

Today, we rarely have the need of fight or flight due to some predator wanting to eat us. We also don't have to hunt and gather for survival. Predators are not chasing most of us, nor do we need to walk to the river to find water. We also don't climb trees to pick fruits and berries. We don't squat to go to the bathroom in the outdoors. For thousands of years we did. Survival depended on the proper movement of our body to make it happen.

In modern society, we do not get the consistent movement our bodies are designed for. Convenience of movement has become ingrained in us from the time we were young. We drive cars to go everywhere, whether to get to work or drive for a quick visit to a friend's house down the road. A hundred years ago we were much more likely to walk. Consequently, the lack of walking is hurting the way we move on a daily basis.

Lack of physical stimulus has encouraged a reduction in movement, and convenience in our society has allowed our natural movements to be lost. The reduction of movement in certain areas has caused other areas to compensate. As a result, certain muscles become out of balance as we grow older.

The problems that create chronic pain are not happening because of the way we are designed but, rather, due to the stresses from our environment. Every day's lack of movement is a stimulus that creates tightness in some muscles and weakness in others. Other muscles have to make up for that weakness, which is when compensation occurs. Compensation can be a slow process that happens over time, or if we have a traumatic event like an accident, it can happen quickly.

Movement encourages balance and symmetry and decreases compensation. The more varied the movement, the better it is for the body. Exercises designed to fix your specific compensation issues will allow you to move better, feel younger, and be more active. They will help to stop your compensation and allow your body to move the way it is designed to move.

Let's revisit the car accident example from the discussion on acute pain causing chronic pain. When a client has had a major event like a car wreck, they usually know the reason pretty quickly. But sometimes the reason is not from something so drastic as a car wreck or a major accident; it stems from something like a sprained ankle when they were young or a sports injury in high school.

Once the source of the pain is identified, the next question I often get is, "Why am I moving that way?" Many times I don't know the reason because there could be many possibilities. Getting you to feel better and move better is about changing your current dysfunctional movement patterns. This will allow healing which will make you feel better.

When the injury happened, the body learned to compensate in order to move. This might have happened for several weeks to several months. Compensating for that injury forced the muscles in the affected joints to become tight, which decreased their range of motion. So even after that specific injury healed, the body was never fixed of its compensation. That compensation has created chronic pain years later.

Repetitiveness

Asking your body to do something for long amounts of time is repetitiveness, and repetitive movement is another source of chronic pain. An example of this is a beautician or barber who has to stand for long periods, or like my father who sits for long periods because he drives a semi truck.

I like to use a simple equation to determine how repetitiveness affects the body. The demand of an activity times the amount of time doing that activity equals a positive or negative change in the body.

Demand of Activity x Time Doing the Activity = Positive or Negative Impact on Body

This equation can be applied to how muscles develop and how they move. The human body reacts to stimuli. Positive stimuli to the muscles causes the body to move properly, and negative stimuli to the muscles causes the body to move improperly. The amount of time doing the positive or negative movement can directly affect having or not having chronic pain.

People who stand for long periods, such as beauticians and teachers, illustrate the impact of repetitiveness. They are standing on their feet most of the day, which can put stress on their backs and hips. This stress builds over time. Standing for many years multiplies the demand on the body.

We can also apply this formula to people who have an active lifestyle. They find something they like to do and, thinking it is healthy, they do more of it. Many of my clients are golfers, tennis players, runners and cyclists, and they still have chronic pain because they are doing their favorite activity too much. These activities are great for the body, but overdoing them can actually have a negative impact.

I'm not advocating you stop doing them. I'm implying that if you like to do them, you have to create balance to make sure you can do them without causing harm. Instead of saying don't do them, I'm saying you need to add proper movements somewhere in your daily life that will help you do them better so they don't create pain.

The Golf Example

Golf is a great sport and great activity, especially if you are walking the course. But the repetitiveness of golfing can be detrimental to your body. Doing the same activity over and over again, whether it is golfing, playing tennis, running, or cycling, creates wear on the joints and leads to chronic pain.

I love the saying, "Variety is the spice of life," and how it applies to the human body. The key to being healthy is in the variety of your activities: run, jump, play, and do all kinds of movements and activities. Don't get tunnel vision with one particular sport or one specific workout plan. Mix it up.

What if you can't vary your activity? What if you have a job that requires you to sit for hours a day? What if you love to golf and don't want to do anything else?

THERE IS A SOLUTION: CREATE A POSTURAL BRIDGE

Implementing a postural bridge allows you perform the activities you want to do while countering the negative impact on your body from repetitive motion. The exercises at the end of this book serve as a postural bridge that will help you.

Repetitive Sitting

Let's revisit sitting, this time from the perspective of repetitiveness. Sitting for long periods creates muscular dysfunctions, causing certain muscles in the body to become tight and other muscles to become weak. Muscular imbalance negatively affects how your joints and bones move. Then you apply the amount of time sitting, which multiples the effect it has on the body.

The requirement of the human body to sit has become predominate in the workplace, and we sit for hours and hours. Then it becomes years and years. The actual position of sitting is not bad for short periods of time but the repetitiveness of sitting for long periods is bad for the body.

The Workout Crowd

Working out is good, and it is healthy for you. My goal is to help you work out better, but not by changing what you do or telling you what workout is better than others.

What you take into the workout, you get out of the workout. If you sit all day and then go to the gym, you are taking that sitting position of shoulders rounded and hips tucked into the gym. You are actually reinforcing the sitting position. Taking bad alignment, poor posture, and lack of function into a workout will only exacerbate the issues.

Working out can improve some of the negative effects of sitting, such as blood pressure, hormones and weight issues, but not all of them. If you have a job that involves sitting five to six hours a day, walking on the treadmill for a warm up won't reverse those effects. Working out for an hour is not enough to counteract the multiple hours of negative repetitiveness on your postural muscles caused by the modern day environment you live in.

You don't have to stop working out, but work out better. You have to do something specifically focused on changing your posture and alignment. There needs to be a postural bridge from your sitting position to your working out position to reinforce good function.

As a transition, perform exercises that focus on restoring your body's good posture, muscle balance, and joint alignment before going to the gym. This creates a stronger, better bridge that allows you to do what you love to do and makes your workout more effective and better for your body.

Posture and the Kinetic Chain

Much more than just standing tall or sitting correctly, posture is correctly connecting the top of your body to the bottom so it moves together. It means getting your feet pointed properly and your hips positioned correctly, as well as many other aspects of your body's overall alignment.

As we noted earlier, the kinetic chain is a term from engineering that describes how the bones, joints, connective tissues, and systems work together to produce movement.

The body is a very complicated machine. Our muscles, tendons, and ligaments are the pulleys, belts, and sprockets. Our bones are the supporting structure and foundation. The heart, lungs, veins, and arteries are the fuel, cooling, and hydraulic systems. Looking at how the whole structural machine works is the key to improving chronic pain.

If alignment is the blueprint of the body, the kinetic chain is the chain reaction (or ripple effect) of the blueprint in action.

Looking at your arm, the ulna and radius bones make up the bottom half, and the humerus bone constitutes the upper half. These bones by themselves have no movement. If you try to bend one of these bones, it would break.

But the arm is a kinetic chain that is able to move because we put an elbow joint in the middle. Then we add ligaments and tendons for stability and a few layers of muscles to act as pulleys and levers to cause motion to happen. The nervous system, lymphatic system, and vascular system are all added to aid that movement.

What happens when your kinetic chain is not working properly? Pain!

Let's take a look at the kinetic chain of your leg, starting at your ankle, moving up to your knee, and then into your hip. Then let's say you are having knee pain.

What is the relationship between your knee pain and how your hip and ankle are moving?

Your knee is designed to move like a door hinge. There is very little rotation in your knee joint—rotation happens from your hip. Tight muscles in your hip force the femur, knee, ankle, and foot to point out. When you walk, your knee is bending because you are moving forward—the knee must bend for you to move forward. When your alignment is not correct, the kinetic chain is forced to move improperly, which puts stress on the cartilage, tendons, and ligaments in your knee. The stress from improper movement will break the knee down over time, eventually creating chronic pain.

Improper kinetic chain movement can create issues, but proper kinetic chain movement can fix issues. To make the knee feel better, you must fix how the kinetic chain is operating. To change how the kinetic chain is moving, you must re-educate the muscles that move the chain. You have to get the knee to move as it was designed to move through proper function. When it starts to move as it was designed, the wearing and breaking down will stop. Then the body will start to heal the injured area.

Case Study: Prevent Knee Replacement

Several years ago, Richard, a client who was in his 50s came into my office with severe knee pain. Every step he took was painful. He couldn't climb stairs without pain. He couldn't do much of anything because his knee would hurt too much when any kind of stress was placed on it. Even such little demand as walking from his living room to his kitchen hurt it.

Before coming into the clinic, he went to the doctor, who took an X-ray and showed him how the painful knee was "bone on bone."

The doctor suggested he should live with the pain as long as he could, and when the pain was so bad he couldn't stand it, he should have the knee replaced. Richard wasn't very happy with that approach, and when he asked for alternatives, the doctor offered shots and pain meds.

Like most of my clients, he had heard about me from a friend who had seen success through the program. After a thorough evaluation and several visits, his knee was feeling much better—to the point that it no longer hurt when walking and created no problem going up stairs. He was back to leading a normal active life.

Unfortunately, his daughter broke her arm, which led him back to the same doctor who had diagnosed his knee. While getting X-rays of his daughter's arm, the doctor suggested he get an X-ray of his knee to see how badly it had degenerated over the past year.

In bewilderment, the doctor showed him the X-rays and congratulated him on preventing his knee replacement. The cartilage seemed to have grown back, and he no longer had a knee that was bone on bone.

I did not give him some magic exercise for his knee. During his evaluation, I had noticed his hip was not moving correctly. The incorrect movement of his hip forced his femur and knee to move medially (inward) with each step. We taught his hip to move correctly, which decreased the wearing on his knee and allowed less breaking down of his cartilage, thus stopping the pain.

After the first diagnosis from his doctor, Richard took it upon himself to find a better solution for dealing with his issues. He was proactive in his search for better answers. The same goes for you; you must be proactive and take control of your body and your health. Pain does not go away by sitting around waiting for it to go away. You have to take action to feel better and move better.

CHAPTER 4
The Pain-Free Life Program

The Pain-Free Life Program is a whole body approach that uses corrective exercises and corrective exercise positions to restore your body's posture and alignment to its original blueprint. When your body is closer to the designed blueprint, you move more efficiently. By addressing your entire body's biomechanics—not just the areas where you have chronic pain—we eliminate continual wear and tear on your joints, reduce the associated pain and inflammation, and allow your body to heal.

Good posture, alignment, and balance are obtained through proper muscle activation. Muscle stimulation comes from strengthening and stretching. General strengthening and stretching are good, but the more specific you can make exercise routines for your issues and your body's imbalances, the better.

Think of all exercises ever created and put them into a large funnel. At the top of the funnel are the general exercise routines that are good for the heart and lungs and help you lose weight. As you move down the funnel, the exercises get more specific. At the bottom of the funnel, exercises are designed specifically for your body and are corrective movements and positions unique to your issues and muscle dysfunctions.

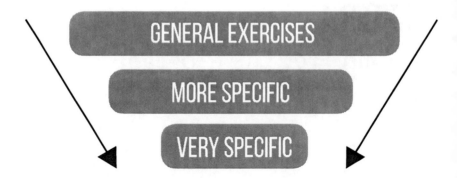

The Pain-Free Life Program concentrates on the exercises at the bottom of the funnel so that the exercises at the top of the funnel work better for you.

Using exercise to fix chronic pain is not a new concept. There have been varying forms and approaches throughout history. Yoga has been around for centuries. They might not call it postural therapy, but if movement helps function, then yoga is helping your posture through better function. Joseph Pilates developed a form of postural therapy in the 1930s, when he designed exercises to create strength and flexibility. Dancers and athletes all over the world have adopted his methods.

As the chronic pain epidemic grows, more physical therapists and personal trainers are adapting their specialized therapies and programs to incorporate postural alignment techniques in addressing their clients' issues. They know the concept, understand it, and realize that a majority of their clients need postural help. Many of these practitioners are some of my biggest client referral sources.

What sets the Pain-Free Life Program apart from these other exercise programs is that it is entirely focused on chronic pain—and that's what makes it so successful. It is a system of implementing the proper movements and positions to achieve the optimum success that your body can achieve. It gets your body to function better so you can move better, allowing you to be active and feel better.

When I first started working with people who had chronic pain, saying that changing posture would fix pain was an outrageous idea. While I have seen a real turnaround in many medical practitioners' thoughts on posture and the effect on chronic pain, there still needs to be a major paradigm shift in the way we address chronic pain rehabilitation in our society. That shift needs to start with you.

The Positive Side Effects

Feel Younger

Clients often express how much younger they feel after going through the program. When their posture is better on a consistent basis, they don't have chronic daily physical problems. They often report that their friends have commented on how they have become more energized and how good they look. More energy leads to being more active and staying active throughout your life. Study after study has scientifically proven that being active makes you feel younger. A body aligned through structural muscle education functions properly and is the first stepping-stone to feeling better and being more active.

Unfortunately, getting older is unavoidable. But the negative effects of age on your body can be slowed down, which can make you feel younger than you feel right now.

Often an event in your life triggers the quick downward spiral of aging—you throw your back out, or you do something that hurts your knee; it can be anything that forces you to slow down, such as a pulled muscle or joint replacement. Your body never seems to fully recover from that event, which limits your movements and then limits your life. The pain builds and builds leading to pain medications and surgeries.

You can prevent the downward spiral from happening. Even if you have already been through the surgeries and are currently taking the pain medications, you can change. You can feel younger and move better than you do right now. It is just a matter of taking that first step toward better health.

The saying "over the hill" brings to mind getting to the top of the hill one day, and then plunging downhill in an unstoppable crash to your death. Instead of it being a tumbling rockslide that nothing can stop, how about making the hill just a speed bump and growing old gracefully?

Imagine if you could reverse the feeling of being old. What would you feel like being young again, hiking mountains, going for a long walk, or getting on the floor to play with your grandkids? How would you feel not having to worry about getting back up from the floor because your knee or back hurt, or about the side effects of pain when you did?

Eliminate Osteoporosis

Phyllis was told at the age of 60 that she had the bones of a 90-year-old. She followed her doctor's recommendations of doing weight bearing exercises and taking the prescribed medications; yet follow-up tests showed that her bone density was getting worse instead of better.

In her search for help, she read an article about how better posture can help decrease osteoporosis. As she researched more on the subject, she soon became convinced that her bad posture and alignment was creating her declining bone density.

She eventually found her way to my office, where she started her journey toward better posture and alignment. At her next osteoporosis checkup, she was told to keep doing what she was doing because her bone density age was 10 years younger than her original scan.

Because we live on Earth, we always have the force of gravity pulling on our bodies. As we grow older, gravity starts to have a bigger effect; we start to round our shoulders, and our back starts to hunch over. When we realize this is happening, we go to the doctor and ask why we are starting to look like an elderly person. The doctor's typical reply is, "You have osteoporosis." Age is often blamed for osteoporosis, but if that were true, then every person over a certain age would have it.

The Mayo Clinic says, "Bone is living tissue that is constantly being broken down and replaced. Osteoporosis occurs when the creation of new bone doesn't keep up with the removal of old bone." The recommendations by the Mayo Clinic for preventing or improving osteoporosis are a healthy diet, weight-bearing exercises, and medication.

According to ConsumerReports.org, research has found that bisphosphonates (medications prescribed by doctors for osteoporosis) offer only modest benefits in building bone and preventing fractures. All pose risks, and growing evidence has now linked the drugs to "a long list of worrisome side effects."

Even more concerning, many doctors have started prescribing bisphosphonates not just for people with osteoporosis but also for those with osteopenia, or pre-osteoporosis, even though the drugs' effectiveness are less clear for this more common condition.

What if there was a natural way to prevent osteoporosis or a natural way to correct it without medications and all their malevolent side effects?

No matter your age, your body still has the ability to heal. I tell my clients that if you can still breathe, you can still heal. The healing process might not be as fast as it was when you were 18 years old, but even at 100 years old, your body is still

SIDE EFFECTS OF OSTEOPOROSIS MEDICATIONS

Increased Joint Pain
Severe Musculoskeletal Pain
Hypocalcemia (too little calcium in blood)
Throat Cancer
Atrial Fibrillation
Bone Fractures
Constipation
Diarrhea
Headaches
Swelling of Hands and Feet

making new cells. You can drastically improve or even eliminate osteoporosis, because you have the ability to heal.

Weight-bearing exercise is not enough. Pulling your shoulders back when working out is not enough. You have to have a better bridge into your weight-bearing exercises. You have to have the proper spine, hip, and shoulder alignment while doing them in order to see desired improvement. You have to get the deep structural muscles to do their jobs and teach the muscles to move the bones into proper alignment naturally. Only when you are consistently aligned and function properly will you see the reverse and eventual stop of osteoporosis.

Flexibility, Strength, and Balance

Being functional is essential to reducing pain and feeling younger.

"Functional" is the term I use to describe someone who is strong and flexible with proper range of motion. Being functional is the combination of three elements: flexibility, strength, and balance. You should be flexible but not too flexible, and you should be strong but not too strong. You need to be in balance to be functional.

Often clients notice one side of their bodies is tighter than the other. This imbalance can come from overusing one side, which is the result of the body compensating for a weakness. When this happens, a twofold approach is applied to create balance: when a specific muscle is stretched, you must strengthen its opposing muscle group also, so that it can hold the stretched position longer and more consistently.

As we grow older, our function decreases because our flexibility or our strength decreases. Muscles, tendons, and ligaments naturally get tighter and less elastic as you grow older. Symptoms of decreased function are frequent cramping, "charley horses" in the muscles, or stiffness in the joints or low back when you wake up in the morning.

Because flexibility affects your daily movement, flexibility relates directly to function. If you can't bend over to tie your shoes because of tightness, you have lost function as a result of your lack of flexibility. If you can't cross your leg on your knee to put your socks on, your lack of flexibility has caused you to lose function. Decrease of function limits movement of your joints, which wears and breaks them down.

But I also want to warn that being flexible is not the only concern if you have tight muscles. To feel better and have less pain, you need to be functional, not just flexible. If you have had tight muscles for many years, those tight muscles have also created weak muscles. Because your muscles work as a group, not individually, one tight muscle affects other muscles. I see this often when I work on yoga participants. They have amazing flexibility, but their alignment is off. They are not functioning properly, which creates pain.

Case Study: Strength Is Not the Solution

On a therapy trip to Atlanta several years ago, I worked with a client who was having back pain. As we were going through the evaluation process, I asked him why he thought he was having pain.

His response was that he thought he was very weak, and by his reasoning, he thought he should start lifting weights again to stop his pain. Several years prior, he began having back pain, and the pain went away when he began working out at the gym. He had quit working out since then, and his back pain was worse than ever.

Another therapist was working on a client across the room who I knew was there because of back pain. The other therapist's client was an NFL lineman—a very big guy who was around 6'7", lean, and muscular. As part of the evaluation process with the other therapist, the professional football player had his shirt off. I could tell by looking at him that he could probably bench press me a dozen times and then throw me out the window.

When my client had told me about his theory of fixing back pain, I replied, "Take a look at that guy across the room. Can you guess why he is here?" My client said he had no idea, because the guy looked pretty healthy.

I told him the other client was there because he has been having back pain. Then I asked my client if he thought he lifted weights? "Well, I think that's pretty clear," my client replied. I guarantee that an NFL lineman lifts weights, yet he was struggling with the same problem as my client.

To alleviate pain and help you feel younger, the Pain-Free Life Program addresses better flexibility, strength, and balance by focusing on the specific muscles impacting your body as a whole.

When you are functional, you feel better. When you feel better, you are more active. Doing the things you love to do without pain makes you feel better and younger. Feeling better is a cycle, and one thing leads to the next. There is no magic pill or potion, but there is a process of getting the correct elements in place that will allow your body to feel younger.

Sleep and Stress

One of the questions most asked by clients with back pain is about their mattress. I don't think mattresses cause back pain—your body's misalignment and dysfunction cause back pain. The mattress might facilitate a position that puts pressure on your back, but issues with your body are creating the pain.

Many of us have heard stories of people with back pain buying new mattresses and their pain going away. But inevitably the pain will be back. They have to fix their body, not just change their environment.

The sleeping hours are not causing pain; at night your body is calming down. The rate at which your heart is pumping slows down, which is decreasing the amount of blood that is being distributed through your body. Muscles are trying to relax, which can cause instability. The instability causes pain.

Something is going on while you are awake that is stressing your back, but you might not feel it until you are lying in bed, or when you get out of bed in the morning.

If you can't sleep because you have pain, your ability to manage stress will be affected. If you are tired and sleepy throughout your day, your stress levels will increase dramatically. You have to be proactive to fix the problem causing the pain. When you fix your pain, you can get more sleep.

Common sense says that sleep and stress affect each other. When you search Google for studies on sleep and stress, you get about 1.7 million results. There is a connection.

If chronic pain is keeping you up at night, your ability to manage stress will be negatively impacted. Sometimes it feels like an endless cycle with one negative affecting the other. There needs to be something that interrupts the negative cycle. Often that interruption can be focusing on improving your posture and function.

I also get asked, "What sleeping position is best?" I don't have an answer, because I don't think there is a specific position every person should be sleeping in to prevent back pain. Everyone is different. The most important point is that you get sleep; positioning doesn't really matter, provided you are comfortable.

I have worked with clients who have had such extreme pain that the only sleeping position comfortable is in a recliner. If I told them to sleep in a bed because sleeping in a recliner is bad, they would not to be able to sleep because of pain. The goal is to get them comfortable in a bed, but that change happens during the waking hours, not the sleeping hours. The sleeping position is not the concern; the body's alignment affecting the sleeping position is.

Brain Power

Everybody knows that exercise is good for you, and if you need convincing of that, you are probably reading the wrong book. Exercise increases blood flow, directly affects the chemicals in the brain that create new brain cells, and helps the current brain cells survive longer. Exercise also improves insulin resistance, reduces inflammation, and stimulates positive factors for proper brain growth.

But what if you can't exercise because you have pain? What if the activity is something you love to do? Some people will battle through the pain, ignoring it the best they can. Others will avoid the activity causing the pain altogether.

Fixing the source of pain allows you to do whatever you love to do, without limitations. To begin, you need to create a solid foundation in your body. That foundation is good posture and good alignment.

Every year the scientific community is learning more and more about the human body. Yet we still know very little about how a lot of systems within our body actually work. We know exercise is good for us, but how good is it? Can it reverse disease? Can it reverse the aging process? Can it fix chronic pain?

Researchers at the University of Kansas Medical Center are studying the effects of exercise in preventing Alzheimer's disease. However, the complexity of the brain makes understanding the effects of exercise on it difficult, so studies about Alzheimer's disease take years to accomplish.

In a New York Times article, Gretchen Reynolds wrote, "Just how exercise remakes minds on a molecular level is not yet fully understood, but research suggests that exercise prompts increases in something called brain-derived neurotropic factor, or B.D.N.F., a substance that strengthens cells and axons, fortifies the connections among neurons, and sparks neurogenesis." A study cited in that article also showed how a group of people who were assigned a walking routine actually demonstrated signs of a younger brain.

The medical community has guesses as to why that happens, but the complexity of the brain makes proving how it happens very hard. They have the proof it helps; they just don't know why it helps.

Being unable to move properly because you have pain will affect your brain. Through the Pain-Free Life Program, you can improve how your body functions in order to move better and feel better. This will translate into helping your brain function better. Start with your alignment and function to create a good foundation, so the environment your body is in can allow your mind to flourish.

---

[2]http://www.nytimes.com/2012/04/22/magazine/how-exercise-could-lead-to-a-better-brain.html?_r=5&pagewanted=all

CHAPTER 5
What It Takes

Reaching the goal of fixing your chronic pain forever and getting back to the active lifestyle you were designed to live takes consistent work. In 20 years of working with clients who have chronic pain, I have found that consistent improvement happens over time. To feel better, you have to work at it every day.

Earlier, we described the downward spiral of health due to chronic pain. Focusing on proper alignment and muscle balance can reverse that process. When you change the way you move, you can live your life without the fear of limitations that stem from chronic pain.

As you re-educate your muscles through corrective positions and postural movements, the momentum starts to change. You start to feel better because you have less pain. You become even more active, and you go for a walk. Over time, you start to feel even better, so you start to jog.

Since you have taught your muscles to move your joints in a healthier way, you are able to increase your activity, which increases your strength and range of motion. Eventually, the downward cycle is halted, and a positive healthy trend has developed that you can maintain consistently throughout your life.

And we know that the healthier you are, the younger you feel. The younger you feel, the happier you are. Not only can you get back the active lifestyle that is good for you, but you can also be better at it than you were before. How is this applied in your favorite activities?

For golfers, you will be able to swing the golf club without pain, and you will have better range of motion that allows you to hit the ball further and more accurately.

For runners, you will be able to run more efficiently, which will allow you to run faster and longer without fatigue and with fewer demands on your joints.

What if you like tennis, yoga, gardening, or you would just like to take the dog for a walk?

The activity doesn't matter; by changing the way you move, you will make the activity good for you instead of a source of pain.

Important Ingredients

In the recipe for fixing chronic pain and limiting the negative effects of modern-day living, two of the most important ingredients are commitment and time. The exercises are the tools you use to reach your goals of having better posture, better alignment and proper function, but the exercises will not work unless you put the effort and time into doing them.

From my many years of working with clients, I also believe

that hope, determination, and a positive attitude are key ingredients for eliminating pain and feeling better. There is no magic pill or magic surgery. If you do the work, you must do it with hope, determination, and a positive attitude. If you are not willing to do the work, you won't feel better.

Commitment and Time

There is no magic exercise. The Pain-Free Life Program guides you but your commitment to the process and dedication is what makes you feel better.

Clients who see the most success are the ones who make a long-term commitment to get better. They work their exercises into their daily routine and get re-evaluated on a regular basis.

When my clients come in for their first visit, the majority of them feel better immediately. However, after the first visit, I warn them that the pain will probably come back. As soon as they drive home and get back to their normal routine, their body will resume its old ways—powered by years of incorrect muscle memory—bringing the pain right back.

They do the routine the next day and feel a little better; maybe the pain stays away a little longer. After performing the routine daily for a few weeks, the pain has gotten noticeably better. They return for a new set of exercises that builds on the first set. The alignment of their body keeps improving, and they get stronger and more balanced.

Depending on the original issues, many feel good enough to go for a walk after they finish their daily routine. These walks will help reinforce healing because the clients are walking with better balance and better alignment.

As you start to feel better and move better on a consistent basis, the need for regular re-evaluations decreases. But unless you quit your job to become a hunter and gatherer, you will always need to do something to counteract the negative effects of today's way of life on your body.

If you analyze the life of an average person, you will see a very sedentary lifestyle. Even people who work out on a daily basis have a sedentary life compared to our hunting and gathering ancestors. The amount of time you have been bombarding your body with negative stimuli directly influences how much wearing and breaking down of your body has occurred.

Walking

For many thousands of years, walking was the way we were able to get from point A to point B. When early humans wanted a drink of water, they had to walk to the stream, or if they were hungry, they had to walk to find their food. Walking is in our DNA. Walking helps the systems of the body function better. The human body is designed to be able to walk without putting excessive pressure on our joints.

Walking is one of the best movements you can do for your body. Yet we are consistently hearing how walking creates issues. The issues are not coming FROM the walking but via the WAY you are walking. The negative influences of our environment have created a dysfunctional body that is trying to move. Moving under the influence of dysfunction will create pain. Fix your dysfunction, and your walking will change.

I recommend to all my clients that they walk more. But what if walking hurts?

POSTURAL BRIDGE = BETTER WALKING

If your body is unable to function properly, then walking can be detrimental for you. Create a better bridge, so that your walking is good for you. Change how you walk through proper muscle education and proper function. Do your exercise routine before you walk, so that you walk better.

How Does Time Create Dysfunction?

A building has layers of beams and support structures to keep it upright. The body has layers of muscles to do the same and help us move without falling over. Deep structural muscles are specialized in moving and stabilizing your structure.

Trying to be as efficient as possible in the output of energy, the human body will use the least amount of muscle fiber engagement to perform an activity. For example, when the body picks up a lightweight object, like a shoe off the floor, it uses only a few muscle fibers. The object doesn't weigh much, so your body expends the bare minimum amount of energy to lift it. However, when the body lifts a heavy item, it will recruit more muscles fibers and other muscles to help get the task done.

When a muscle can't do its job because of weakness or tightness, the body will compensate by recruiting other muscles to help get the work done. Your body likes to recruit bigger muscles to help the smaller, deep structural muscles do their jobs. The more this happens, the weaker the smaller muscles become, thus creating instability in the joints.

If called upon consistently, these larger muscles will establish a pattern of dysfunction by jumping in automatically. Over time, the dysfunctional pattern becomes ingrained through muscle memory. This incorrect muscle memory is the direct cause of wear and inflammation in the joints.

The Journey to Dysfunction

Earlier, we discussed sitting from a repetitiveness perspective, now let's view it in the context of time.

You began your journey of incorrect muscle memory at an early age. Starting in pre-school, you were taught to sit for longer and longer stretches of time. Through elementary school, middle school and high school, you were sitting in class the majority of the day. Then you sat through your college lectures before walking to the library or your dorm to sit and study. After that, you got a job where you likely sat for long hours, bent over a computer keyboard. You have been training your body to sit for many years.

There are two basic elements to physical health. One element focuses on keeping your heart, lungs, and weight healthy; the other is your body's alignment and posture. Even though the two elements are interconnected, most people ignore the alignment and posture aspect.

People try to counter the years of sitting by going to the gym. They hope that by working out they will improve their posture or their pain. Unfortunately, they are wrong; working out does not prevent chronic pain or fix it. It might delay chronic pain and even reduce it (if you're lucky), but the barrage of negative stimuli from a dysfunctional environment is still there. Lifting weights, yoga class, Pilates class, or spinning classes build upon your body's current dysfunction. They do not retrain your body to function properly in your negatively influenced postural surroundings.

Exercise, as we call it in today's society, has an element of movement. We obviously move when we're on the treadmill or in the pool, but exercise does not incorporate enough structural movement to keep our body aligned and fully functional. Often when you exercise, the bigger outer layers of muscles do more work and overpower the smaller muscles. Taking a misaligned, overcompensated body to the gym can lead to disaster.

The Pain-Free Life Program assesses your body's current dysfunction, then re-educates how you move, so that you can take a better foundation into your exercise classes or workout.

Breaking Habits

The Pain-Free Life Program is a process designed to change how your muscles move your bones. It's a system of re-education for the deep structural muscles, which are hard to isolate, so that they can break out of the habitual patterns that have moved your joints improperly for years (even decades in some cases).

We interrupt this pattern and introduce proper stimuli to create positive muscle memory. Muscle education is stimulus. The goal is to get more positive stimuli than negative stimuli to your muscles.

Just as your body took time to establish incorrect muscle memory patterns, your body will need time to correct them. While the re-education process takes time, it is one you can—and should—start right away. The exercises at the end of this book give you something that you can do at home to start re-educating these muscles.

Healing

As mentioned throughout this book, here at Exercise Therapy of Kansas City we focus on the physical aspects of chronic pain: fixing posture, alignment, and dysfunction to create an environment in which your body will feel better. But I would not be totally truthful if I left out some other very important aspects that I have found also contribute to putting an end to your chronic pain.

Hope, Determination, and a Positive Attitude

I recently read about Master Sergeant Raul (Roy) Benavidez. He was a member of the United States Army Special Forces who received the Medal of Honor for his actions in the Vietnam War.

While at the hospital, suffering from the many ramifications of a mine exploding under him, he was told that he would never walk again. He said he was stunned by the diagnosis and refused to believe it—and was determined to prove them wrong.

About his diagnosis, Benavidez said:

"Declared never to walk again, the doctors were preparing my medical discharge papers. But at night I would slip out of bed and crawl to the wall. Using my elbows and chin, my back would be killing me, I would be crying…I would remember in my special forces training, on one of the training missions I was on, my leader would tell me, faith, determination, and a positive attitude will carry you further than ability. He would say, 'You can do it Benavidez, you can do it.' I never forgot those words, never…Nine months later I was able to walk out of that hospital."

Three years later, he would find himself again near death from gunshot and stab wounds inflicted while helping a surrounded patrol. From his medical reports after the event, Benavidez had a total of 37 separate bullet, bayonet, and shrapnel wounds from the six-hour fight with an enemy battalion.

During Benavidez' Medal of Honor speech in 1991, Ronald Reagan described his heroic endeavors:

"Prior to reaching the team's position he was wounded in his right leg, face, and head. Despite these painful injuries, he took charge, repositioning the team members and directing their fire to facilitate the landing of an extraction aircraft, and the loading of wounded and dead team members. He then threw smoke canisters to direct the aircraft to the team's position.

---

[3]Here is a link to Reagan's speech, award Benavidez's the Medal of Honor and Benavidez's acceptance speech: https://www.youtube.com/watch?v=_oUtJxE4sjs.

Despite his severe wounds and under intense enemy fire, he carried and dragged half of the wounded team members to the awaiting aircraft. He then provided protective fire by running alongside the aircraft as it moved to pick up the remaining team members. As the enemy's fire intensified, he hurried to recover the body and classified documents on the dead team leader."

Master Sergeant Benavidez could have easily given up while lying in his bed three years prior to his heroic actions. He could have taken his discharge papers and retired from the military, never to walk again. But he never gave up; with faith, determination, and a positive attitude, he became a hero.

We can learn a lesson from this great man: anything can be overcome, if we set our mind to it. I see this every day with clients who come in with knee, back, or some other kind of chronic pain.

The clients who get better never give up. They keep an open mind and are focused on getting better. They are not looking for the quick fix but for everlasting pain relief. They have the three factors that Master Sergeant Benavidez had: hope, determination, and a positive attitude.

Hope

If you are in despair from years of chronic pain, hope is a belief that there is the possibility of feeling better. And you hold on to hope that your life will get better. Hope can be the life-saving rope keeping you from falling further into the abyss of despair and leading you to feeling good again. You just have to climb it hand-over-hand until you gain solid ground.

Clients come in to the clinic searching because they know, deep down inside, there are better answers to helping their pain. They know they don't have to live with those dire diagnoses as labels.

Having hope that there is a path to feeling better, you will find what answers you believe are best for you. You are being proactive in your healing and not taking a backseat to your diagnoses. Believe you are taking responsibility for getting yourself better. You are in charge of your body. Focus on the possibility of becoming pain-free.

The feeling of hope that you can fix your pain may wax and wane from day to day. It is like a rollercoaster with ups and downs. One day you feel you are really making progress, and a week later, you feel all is lost. The path to becoming pain-free is a process. Depending on the level of pain and your specific issues, the path is usually not a quick fix. However, baby steps will eventually turn into giant steps.

The exercises you find at the end of this book are the first steps to regaining that solid ground. They are the first steps to transforming you into a more active, healthier person.

Determination

Determination is the proactive step. With hope you believe in yourself that you can improve your chronic pain. Determination is putting the process in motion: doing what you need to do on a consistent basis which means doing your routine daily.

Determination is action.

Some clients, when they first come in, have reached the end of their rope. They have tried everything, and nothing has worked. They feel they are cursed, or there is nothing they can do to feel better.

I encourage them to keep moving forward and not give up, to be determined in the fight to feel better.

Clients who see the most success are those who are determined to do so through the ups and downs. They do their exercises daily. They are determined to do the things that are going to get them better. There might be some times of doubt or difficulty, but they fight through with determination.

Feeling better takes time and dedication because we are combating decades of dysfunction. Determination is the key to pushing on when you feel like you just want to stay in bed.

TESTIMONIAL: NED KEHDE

The Pain-Free Life Program has made me virtually pain-free, and when pain does occasionally erupt in my 71-year-old body, Travis creates a series of exercises for me.

I haven't had an aspirin or any pain medication since mid-May of 2009, which was when I was hit hard with some TMJ. At that time he gave me eight exercises that fixed it in two days.

Besides TMJ, in the 10 years I have worked with Exercise Therapy of Kansas City, Travis has helped many other issues that have afflicted me. I rarely miss a day of doing my routine. His program helps keep me active as I grow older. I feel better now than when I was in my 50s.

Positive Attitude

Having a positive attitude when things are going well is easy; being positive during the trying times can be difficult. If you are having debilitating chronic pain, you know how hard having a positive attitude can be. Even having minor pain can adversely affect your attitude, especially if it keeps you from doing what you love to do.

When you have pain and you can't do the things you love to do, you start to feel your life is at a standstill. But to feel better you have to have a positive mindset. The best way to have a positive attitude is to be proactive about your life. Whether eating better or exercising consistently, you have to be moving forward to have a positive attitude.

To quote the great Winston Churchill: "Never give in, never, never, never, never—in nothing, great or small, large or petty—never give in…" On the days when your pain level is so bad that you don't want to get out of bed, you have to tell yourself, "This is the day I make one more step toward feeling better; even if the step is small, it is a step in the right direction."

The Story of Clare

Clare came into the clinic with a long history of chronic back pain. Every morning was a struggle for her to get out bed. The physical struggle weighed on her mentally. She felt her life was cursed and this was just the way she was meant to be.

She told me her history of three back surgeries and how none of them helped. Often the surgery would stop one pain but create other. She even elected, through the recommendation of one of her doctors, to get a spinal fusion; again, no success.

The reason most people get a spinal fusion is because of instability of the spine. The typical thought process is that the instability is creating the problem. The thought process is right, but the solution of a spinal fusion is wrong—our spine is meant to move. Decreasing movement where there should be movement leads to other problems. It might stop instability in a specific area but it creates greater stress in other areas.

Muscles stabilize the spine. Muscles move bones. There has to be proper hip alignment, shoulder alignment, and spine alignment in order to stabilize the spine. Muscle education of getting the shoulders, hips, and spine to align will create stability and lead to feeling better.

After six visits, Clare reported that getting out of bed was much, much easier. She also reported that after doing her morning exercise routine she felt good enough to face the day, which led to a better attitude throughout the whole day.

She still has to battle the pain and, due to all she has been through, she might have to for the rest of her life. But compared to the depression and the hopelessness she felt before, she was looking at the world with a better attitude. She overcame that hopelessness and started to believe there was a chance to continually get better.

Chronic pain is not a curse that you have to live with the rest of your life. However, you must be proactive about fixing it; chronic pain is not going to magically disappear. Fixing your chronic pain takes work and time, but what if your efforts relieve your pain by 50 percent? Feeling 50 percent better will be the stepping-stone to feeling 100 percent better.

CHAPTER 6
Corrective Exercises for Your Pain

As I mentioned at the beginning of the book, the goal of the Pain-Free Life Program is to keep you doing what you love to do or get you back to doing what you love to do. Whatever that activity is, I want you to be able to do it and enjoy doing it without the limitations of chronic pain.

The exercises in the following pages are designed to get you started. There is no magic exercise, but the process is important. Each movement or position is designed to build to the next movement or position. Do them to the best of your ability in the order in which I have written them.

Use these exercises to get moving in the right direction and to start the journey toward becoming more active. For some readers, these exercises will be all you need. For others, these will be the first steps to changing years of bad alignment and muscle dysfunction.

Exercises

In this chapter, I'm going to suggest exercises you can do if you are having chronic pain. They are organized by body part, so if you are having back pain, you do the exercises for the back.

You might notice that some of the exercises are not actually working the area where you are having pain. For example, one of the exercises for back pain actually is working your shoulders. This is by design.

I like to emphasize that you know your body better than anybody else. You must listen to your body— this is imperative. Do not ignore what it tells you. If you know from past experience that a certain position causes pain, then don't do that position. Skip it, and move on to the next position.

As you start to feel better over time, you can go back and try that position or movement again to see if it causes less pain. Do not force your body to do something it does not want to do, but, as your body changes and you start to feel better, you should be able to do more with less pain.

Also, focus on your breathing while performing your exercises. Relax your abdominal muscles and try to relax into the stretches or movements.

These exercises are intended to work the smaller, deeper muscles. I tell my clients to use the 80 percent rule. Do your exercises at an 80 percent effort. When asked to squeeze, squeeze 80 percent, not as hard as you can. We want to isolate specific muscles, and, when you squeeze too hard, you will start to compensate by using other/different muscles to do the exercise.

I would also suggest you keep a journal. Write down which exercises feel good and which exercises are difficult to do. Over time, a journal will help you look back at how you have changed. It will also help you to do your exercises on a consistent basis.

Many of you might need additional help. If you find yourself in this situation, call us and we can discuss a plan to get you pain-free and feeling better.

You can find our contact info at *www.exercisetherapykc.com.*

REMEMBER: WE ARE FIXING THE CAUSE OF PAIN AND NOT JUST WORKING ON THE SYMPTOMS.

Exercises for Ankles/Feet Issues

The ankles and feet take on most of the pressure when we stand or walk. They are supporting the weight of the whole body. In our normal and everyday movement, they are the first defense against gravity, which allows humans to be upright. The arch in the foot of a human is designed to help support the body and dissipate any pressure from the weight of the body.

Because our joints do not move independently of each other, what happens in your knees and hips directly affects your ankles and feet. Plantar fasciitis and bone spurs happen because dysfunctional muscles move the bones incorrectly, causing improper wearing of the ankles and feet. When you re-educate the muscles to move that kinetic chain differently, you will decrease the pressure and decrease the wearing on that joint or area.

Hammertoes, bunions, and corns can be signs of issues that are happening somewhere else in the body. These symptoms are signs of misalignment, and your body is trying to compensate for that misalignment. Therefore, with every step you take, your body is overcompensating for improper movement, causing excessive wearing of specific areas on the foot.

Bunions and corns form in response to friction. Corns develop from friction on the foot that is rubbing on the skin more than it should. Bunions form because of improper friction from the way your foot hits the floor and then pushes off. Both of these symptoms can be helped by educating your feet and ankles to move like they are meant to move.

1. Hip Twist

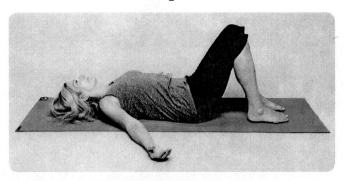

Start by lying on your back. Place your feet hip-width apart with your knees bent at a comfortable angle. When placing your feet hip-width apart, be sure to use the hip joint as reference, not the outside of your hips. You should have your shoulder, hip joint, knees and feet lined up. Place your arms out at your sides at a 45- to 90-degree angle with your palms facing up. Do not place your hands above your shoulders.

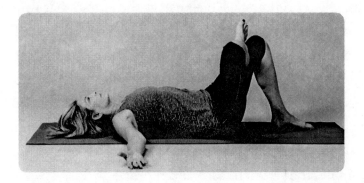

Leaving your left foot on the floor, cross your right ankle over the left knee.

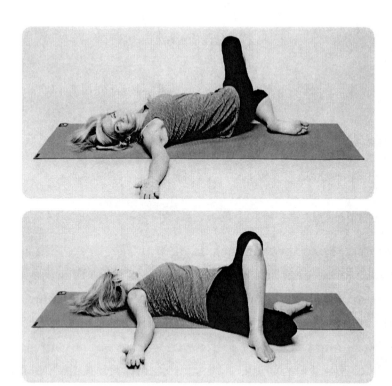

Rotate your right ankle-on-knee to the left, so that your right foot touches the floor. Be sure not to move your left foot; it should only roll to accommodate the rotation. You do not want your left foot to move further away; that would decrease the effect of the exercise. Turn your head to the right. If it is comfortable, press your right knee toward your left foot, opening the hip more, but press only until you feel the stretch. Hold this position for 1 minute, then switch sides and repeat.

2. Assisted Ankle on Knee

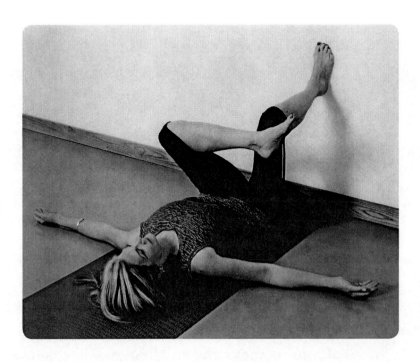

Lie on your back with your feet on the wall. Place your hips far enough away from the wall to create a 90-degree angle in your knees. Place your arms out at your sides at a 45- to 90-degree angle. Place your feet hip-width apart on the wall, using your hip joint as a guide. Then cross your right ankle over your left knee. Press your right knee towards the wall without lifting your butt off the floor. Hold for 1 minute, then switch sides and repeat.

3. Supine Femur Rotations

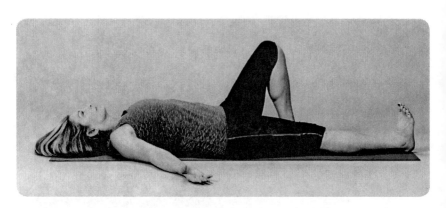

Lie on your back with your knees bent. Place your feet hip-width apart. Place your arms out at your sides at a 45- to 90-degree angle. Extend one leg flat on the floor. Flex the extended leg's foot back, and flex your thigh muscle. Then rotate that leg in and out, creating a windshield wiper movement in your foot. Make the movement happen from your hip muscles. Rotate inward and out as much as you comfortably can. Do not let your hips rotate as you do the movement. Try to focus on the femur bone rotating in the hip socket. Do 30 of the in-and-out movements, then switch sides and repeat.

4. Sitting Knee Pillow Squeezes

Sit on the edge of a chair. Place your feet hip-width apart, with your feet pointed straight ahead. Be sure they do not point out, and be sure they are in line with each other (with the outer sides of the feet parallel). There should be a 90-degree bend in your knees. Roll your hips forward to create a slight arch in your low back. Pull your shoulders back and down, sticking out your chest. Place a block between your knees. You may substitute a small ball for the block. Squeeze the block with your knees. Relax your ab muscles, and remember to breathe. Squeeze the block 60 times, while maintaining the body position.

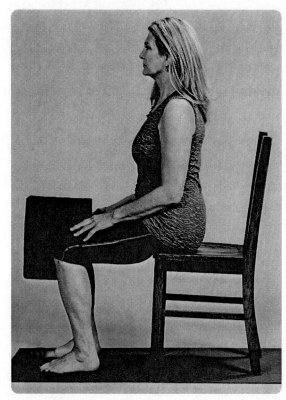

Exercises for Knee Issues

As I mentioned earlier, the knee is like a door hinge, and it is designed to work mainly in extension and flexion. Because it is a part of the kinetic chain, how the muscles move in the hips directly affects the knee. Also affecting the knees are the muscles in the lower leg, such as the calf.

Since the Pain-Free Life Program is designed to work deeper than just addressing the symptom of knee pain, we must look past what the knee is telling us and into what the hips are saying. What is happening with the hips and how they are moving is also going to affect how the knees move and feel.

1. Legs Up Knee Spillow Squeezes

Lie on your back with your knees bent, and place a large block under your legs. You may substitute a chair or coffee table for the block. Keep your knees close to a 90-degree angle while doing this exercise. Place your arms out at your sides at a 45- to 90-degree angle. Place a small block between your knees. Squeeze and release the block with your knees. Be sure not to use your ab muscles while squeezing the block. Keep your ab muscles relaxed, and focus on your breathing as you squeeze. Try to use only your inner thigh muscles. Squeeze 60 times.

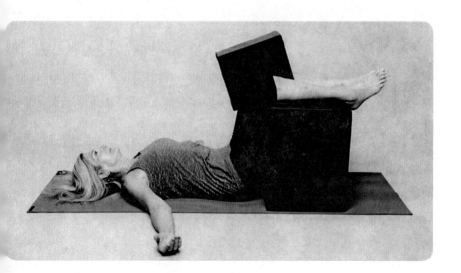

2. Supine Abductor Press

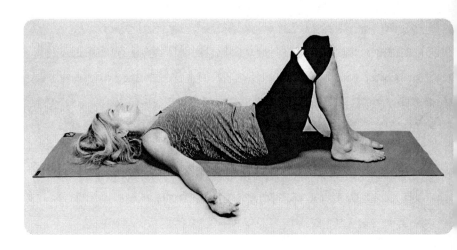

Lie on your back with your knees bent at a comfortable angle. Place your feet hip-width apart, using your hip joint as the reference for your foot position. Place your arms out at your sides at a 45-degree angle. Place a strap around your knees, and tighten the strap so that your knees are slightly less than hip-width apart. Press your legs out against the strap, then release. Do not tighten your abs as you press out. Focus on using the outside of your legs to press out on the strap. Press out and release 60 times.

3. Frog

Start by lying on your back with your legs together, knees bent at a comfortable angle, and feet flat on the floor. Place your arms out at your sides at a 45-degree angle. Relax and let your knees separate and fall toward the floor, putting the soles of your feet together. Hold this position for 1 minute.

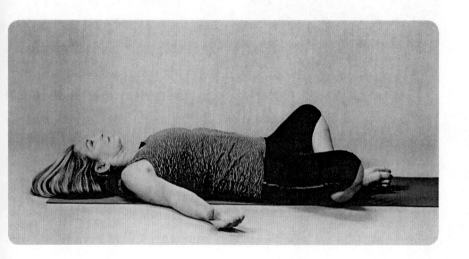

4. Sitting Knee Pillow Squeezes

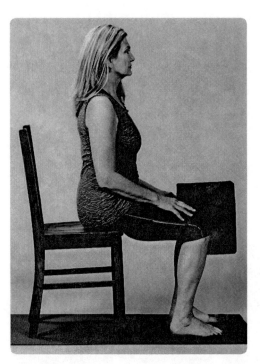

Sit on the edge of a chair. Place your feet hip-width apart, with your feet pointed straight ahead. Be sure they do not point out, and be sure they are in line with each other (with the outer sides of the feet parallel). There should be a 90-degree bend in your knees. Roll your hips forward to create a slight arch in your low back. Pull your shoulders back and down, sticking out your chest. Place a block between your knees. You may substitute a small ball for the block. Squeeze the block with your knees. Relax your ab muscles, and remember to breathe. Squeeze the block 60 times, while maintaining the body position.

Exercises for Hip and Pelvis Issues

The hips and pelvis are the foundation of our spine. Think of the building analogies we have been using throughout this book. In those analogies, the pelvis is the foundation of the building. It is also the major area of our body that creates and directs movement.

When I played sports in high school, the coaches always would tell us not to look at the ball; instead, watch the opposing players' hips to know where they are going. Our hips move our body. Sure, there are other independent movements for fine motor skills or dexterity, but the hips have the biggest and most powerful muscles of our body.

Some of the common symptoms that manifest in the hips are arthritis, bone-on-bone cartilage deterioration in the hip joint, sciatica, and sacroiliac pain (SI pain, as it is commonly called), to name a few. These are all structural issues that can be improved through better alignment and better muscle balance in the hips and pelvic area.

1. Back Extension on Elbows

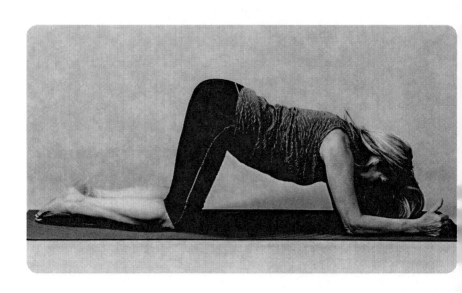

Start on your hands and knees, making sure your hips are directly above your knees and your wrists are directly below your shoulders. Move your hands one hand-length forward, then place your elbows on the floor where your hands were. This should move your hips slightly forward. Roll your hips to create an arch in your low back. Allow your shoulder blades to come together and your chest to fall towards the floor. Hold for 1 minute.

2. Legs Up Wall

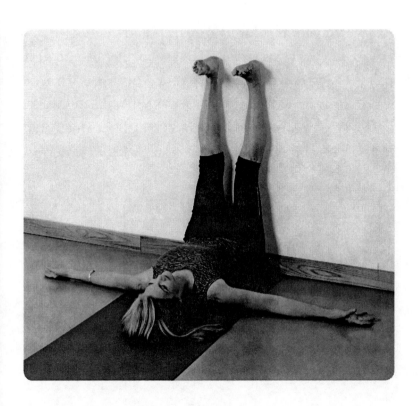

Lie on your back with your legs up the wall. Try to get your butt as close to the wall as possible, while keeping your legs straight. If you can't keep your butt on the floor while your legs are straight, scoot back away from the wall until you can. Pull your toes back and flex your thigh muscles. Try to straighten your legs as much as possible. Keep your feet and knees straight. Do not let your legs roll out. Hold this position for 2 minutes.

3. Standing Arm Circles

Stand with your feet hip-width apart and pointed straight ahead. Extend your arms to the sides at shoulder height with your palms facing down, then move your arms back slightly, just behind your shoulders. Pinch your shoulder blades back and down while sticking out your chest, creating a small arch in your low back. Be sure to keep your hands behind your body. Rotate your arms forward in two-inch circles 40 times. Then, in the same position, turn your palms up, and rotate your arms backwards 40 times.

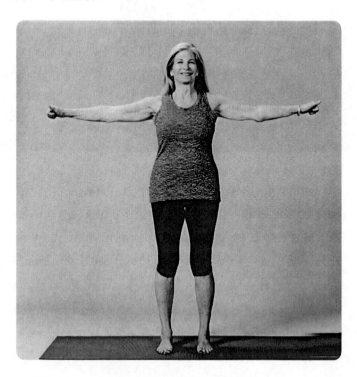

4. Standing Elbow Touches

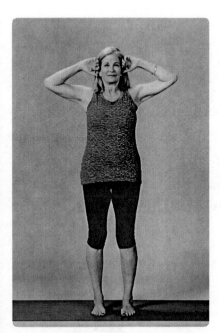 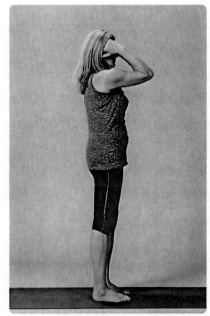

Stand with your feet hip-width apart and pointed straight ahead. Make fists, and place your knuckles on your temples with your thumbs pointing down towards the corners of your mouth. Using your knuckles as hinges, bring your elbows together at shoulder level. Try to keep your head and shoulders lined up while touching your elbows together. Keeping your knuckles on your temples, pull your elbows apart as far back as you comfortably can. Repeat this exercise 30 times.

5. Wall Sit

Stand with your back against a wall. Move your feet away from the wall, keeping them hip-width apart. Begin to slide your hips down the wall until you have reached a sitting position, with an almost 90-degree bend in your knees. Stay slightly above 90 degrees, however. Press your low back into the wall. It is important to keep your ankles in front of your knees and your weight in your heels. This will keep the demand in your quads and not in your knees. Hold for 2 minutes.

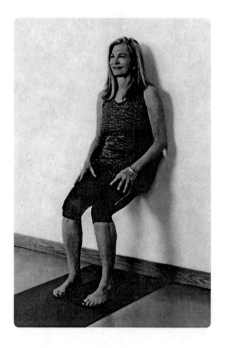
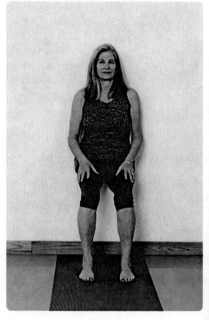

Exercises for Back Issues

The hips and the spine are directly connected. When we take a look at chronic issues of the spine, such as disc herniation, stenosis, bulging disc, slipped disc, degenerated disc disease, and sciatic pain, we also have to look at how the shoulders and the hips work together. The spine helps to connect the hips and the shoulders. It is like a bridge that runs down our body, connecting the upper half to the lower.

If your shoulder position is off, as well as your hip position, then your spine is being drastically affected. That imbalance can create circumstances that cause pain. To fix the pain, you have to get the shoulders and the hips to function properly.

The right and left side should be balanced and mirror each other as closely as possible. When the right and left sides of the pelvis are balanced and the right and left shoulder positions are balanced, then the spine is in an environment which allows it to heal and function better, which means less pain.

1. 90° Legs Up

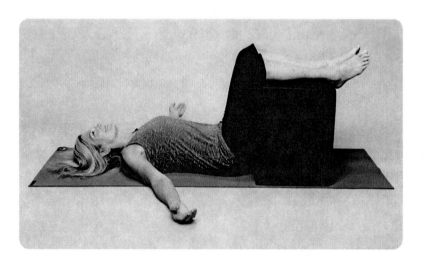

Lie on your back with your knees bent, and place a large block under your legs. You may substitute a chair or coffee table for the block. You want your knees close to a 90-degree angle in this exercise. Place your arms out at your sides at a 45- to 90-degree angle. Let your low back and hips relax into the floor. Take deep breathes from your stomach/diaphragm and not your chest. Stay in this position for 10 minutes.

2. Legs Up Pullover

Lie on your back with your knees bent, and place a large block under your legs. Clasp your hands in the air above you. Pull your hands over your head to the floor. Try to keep your elbows straight but not locked. If you have difficulty getting your hands to the floor, do not force them. Go as far as you can while keeping your elbows straight, and then return your hands to the original position. As you repeat this exercise, you will notice that your hands move closer to the floor. Repeat this movement, down to the floor and back up, 30 times.

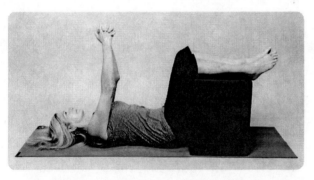

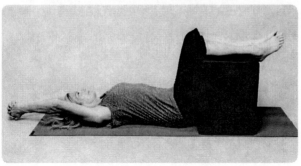

3. Legs Up Knee Pillow Squeezes

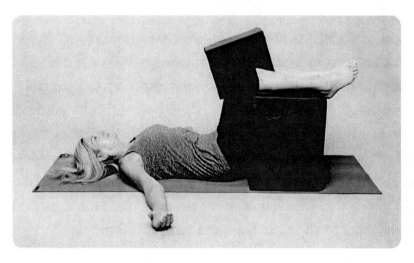

Lie on your back with your knees bent, and place a large block under your legs. You may substitute a chair or coffee table for the block. Keep your knees close to a 90-degree angle while doing this exercise. Place your arms out at your sides at a 45- to 90-degree angle. Place a small block between your knees. Squeeze and release the block with your knees. Be sure not to use your ab muscles while squeezing the block. Keep your ab muscles relaxed, and focus on your breathing as you squeeze. Try to use only your inner thigh muscles. Squeeze 60 times.

4. In and Out's

Lie on your back with your feet on the wall, parallel to each other and more than hip-width apart. Your hips should be away from the wall, so that your knees are at a 90-degree angle. Keeping your feet apart, bring your knees together so they touch. Then spread your knees apart, while rolling your feet out. Try to get your knees as far apart as possible. Then bring them back together. Repeat this motion 30 times.

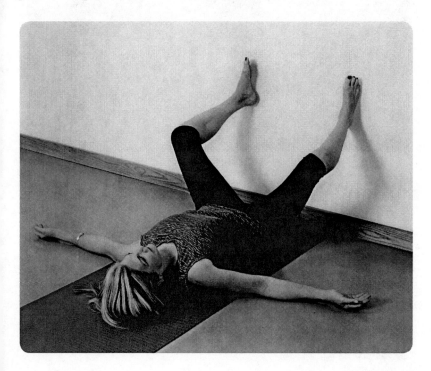

5. Assisted Ankle on Knee

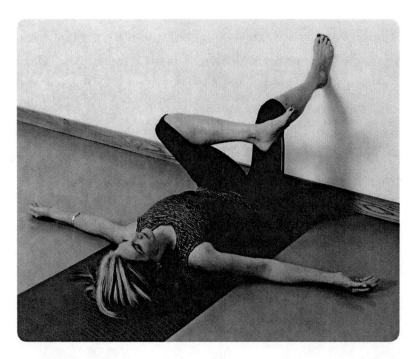

Lie on your back with your feet on the wall. Place your hips far enough away from the wall to create a 90-degree angle in your knees. Place your arms out at your sides at a 45- to 90-degree angle. Place your feet hip-width apart on the wall, using your hip joint as a guide. Then cross your right ankle over your left knee. Press your right knee towards the wall without lifting your butt off the floor. Hold for 1 minute, then switch sides and repeat.

6. Legs Up Wall

Lie on your back with your legs up the wall. Try to get your butt as close to the wall as possible, while keeping your legs straight. If you can't keep your butt on the floor while your legs are straight, scoot back away from the wall until you can. Pull your toes back and flex your thigh muscles. Try to straighten your legs as much as possible. Keep your feet and knees straight. Do not let your legs roll out. Hold this position for 2 minutes.

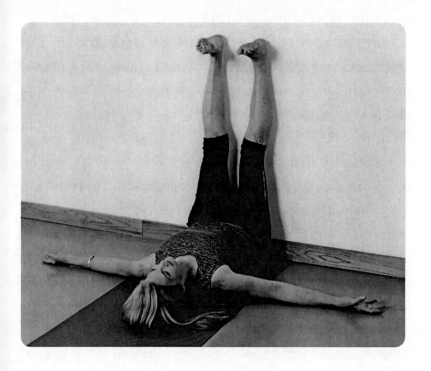

Exercises for Shoulder/Elbow/Wrist Issues

Chronic issues with shoulders, elbows, and wrists often affect people who are very active, like golfers and tennis players. But these issues can affect anyone who has an active or repetitive job, especially where they have to use their hands and arms (such as waitresses, computer users, electricians, and carpenters).

Tendonitis, or tennis elbow, is the inflammation of a tendon in the elbow. Inflammation occurs when that tendon is overused. One solution that the medical field typically suggests is to stop doing that activity. But what if you are an electrician or a carpenter, and you can't quit what you do because you need to feed your family? This also applies to someone who has a desk job and is at a computer for long periods.

Your posture is forcing too much demand from the tendons in your joints. By changing the shoulder blade position, you can create a kinetic chain reaction that eliminates the pressure put on your elbow. The elbow or wrist hasn't created the problem; the rounded position of your shoulder that connects the kinetic chain down your arm has.

When your shoulders are rounded forward, the humerus rotates in the shoulder joint. When your shoulder is in the rounded position for long periods, the muscles attached to the humerus and shoulder joint tighten into that position and decrease in range of motion. From this new "normal" position, moving the joint with an added demand creates pain.

The added demand could be swinging a tennis racket, turning a screwdriver, hammering a nail, or typing on a computer keyboard. Anything that creates repetitive motion can cause chronic pain when the shoulders and the shoulder blades are rounded and not properly functioning.

These exercises will decrease that rounding and allow your elbows, wrists, and hands to function more freely.

1. 90° Legs Up

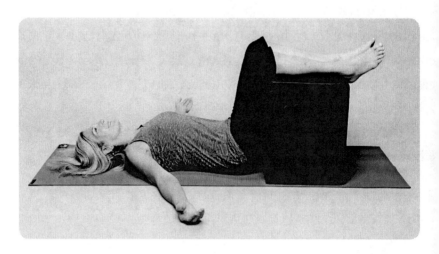

Lie on your back with your knees bent, and place a large block under your legs. You may substitute a chair or coffee table for the block. You want your knees close to a 90-degree angle in this exercise. Place your arms out at your sides at a 45- to 90-degree angle. Let your low back and hips relax into the floor. Take deep breathes from your stomach/diaphragm and not your chest. Stay in this position for 10 minutes.

2. Knee Side to Side

Lie on your back with your knees bent at a comfortable angle, with your feet slightly wider than your hips. Keeping your arms at a 45- to 90-degree angle and your shoulders on the floor, rotate both knees in the same direction as you roll your feet. Try to get the outside knee to the floor. Then rotate your knees to the other side. Do this side-to-side motion 30 times.

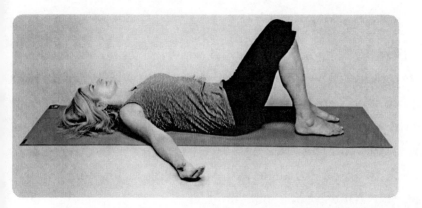

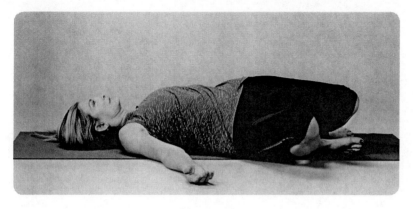

3. Hip Twist

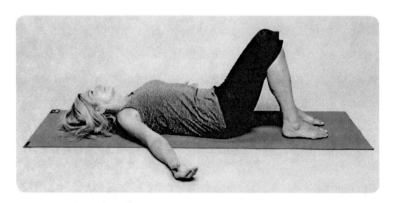

Start by lying on your back. Place your feet hip-width apart with your knees bent at a comfortable angle. When placing your feet hip-width apart, be sure to use the hip joint as reference, not the outside of your hips. You should have your shoulder, hip joint, knees and feet lined up. Place your arms out at your sides at a 45- to 90-degree angle with your palms facing up. Do not place your hands above your shoulders.

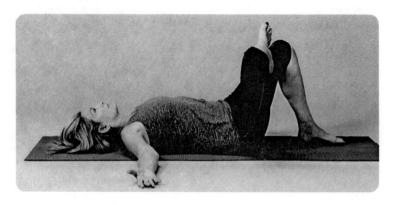

Leaving your left foot on the floor, cross your right ankle over the left knee.

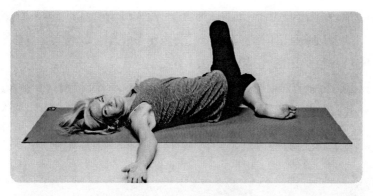

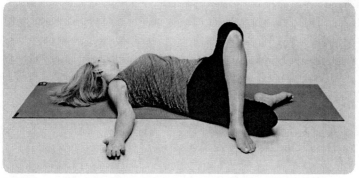

Rotate your right ankle-on-knee to the left, so that your right foot touches the floor. Be sure not to move your left foot; it should only roll to accommodate the rotation. You do not want your left foot to move further away; that would decrease the effect of the exercise. Turn your head to the right. If it is comfortable, press your right knee toward your left foot, opening the hip more, but press only until you feel the stretch. Hold this position for 1 minute, then switch sides and repeat.

4. Cats and Dogs

Move onto your hands and knees. Be sure that your hips are above your knees and your shoulders are above your wrists. Arch your back up, while tucking your head and hips down. Then arch your back down, while lifting your head and sticking your butt up. Breathe out when your back arches up, and breathe in when your back arches down. Move up and down 10 times.

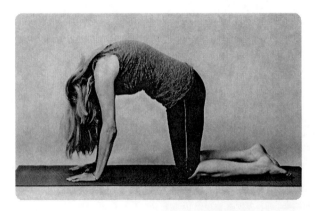

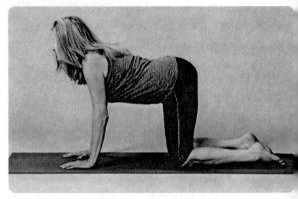

5. Seated Floor

Sit up against a wall. Your butt should be as close to the wall as possible. Flex your feet back, and extend your legs straight. Try to flex your thigh muscles, pushing the backs of your knees to the floor. Keeping your butt and head against the wall, pull your shoulder blades back and down. Hold this position for 2 minutes.

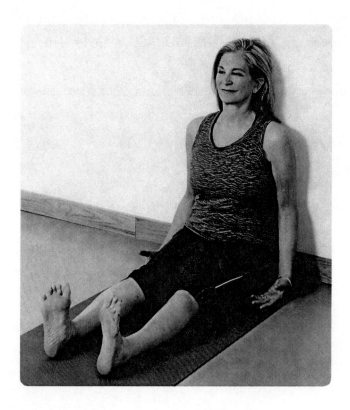

Exercises for Neck and Head Issues

Imagine a bobble-head doll with the head of the doll just nodding away on top of the body. In a very simple way this is what should be happening with your head. The neck muscles are there to support movement and help with balancing the head on the neck.

When the head is not balanced correctly, issues such as TMJ, chronic headaches, migraines, bulging discs, and pinched nerves can occur. To restore balance, all of the load-bearing joints have to line up: hips, shoulders, and neck.

These exercises will help to balance your head on your shoulders and relieve pressure from overuse of the neck and shoulder muscles.

1. 90° Legs Up

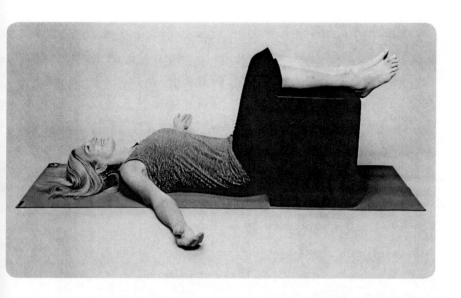

Lie on your back with your knees bent, and place a large block under your legs. You may substitute a chair or coffee table for the block. You want your knees close to a 90-degree angle in this exercise. Place your arms out at your sides at a 45- to 90-degree angle. Let your low back and hips relax into the floor. Take deep breathes from your stomach/diaphragm and not your chest. Stay in this position for 10 minutes.

2. Legs Up Pullovers

Lie on your back with your knees bent, and place a large block under your legs. Clasp your hands in the air above you. Pull your hands over your head to the floor. Try to keep your elbows straight but not locked. If you have difficulty getting your hands to the floor, do not force them. Go as far as you can while keeping your elbows straight, and then return your hands to the original position. As you repeat this exercise, you will notice that your hands move closer to the floor. Repeat this movement, down to the floor and back up, 30 times.

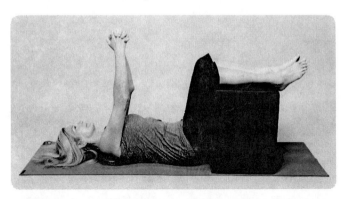

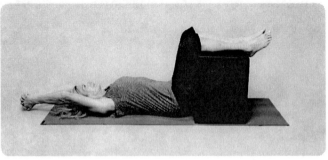

3. Legs Up Scap Presses

Lie on your back with your knees bent, and place a large block under your legs. Place your elbows on the floor at shoulder height with your hands in the air. When you look to the right and left, your elbows should be even. Bend your arms so you have a 90-degree bend in the elbows. Pinch your shoulder blades back and down, and then release. You should not be pressing the elbows into the floor. Focus on your shoulder blades pinching together, then relaxing. Do 30 repetitions.

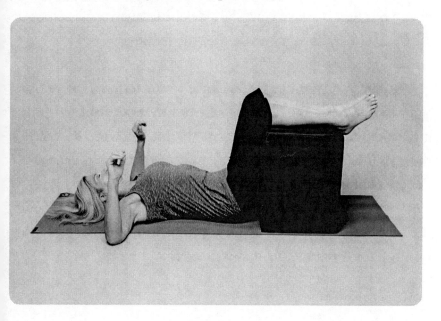

4. Hip Twist

Start by lying on your back. Place your feet hip-width apart with your knees bent at a comfortable angle. When placing your feet hip-width apart, be sure to use the hip joint as reference, not the outside of your hips. You should have your shoulder, hip joint, knees and feet lined up. Place your arms out at your sides at a 45- to 90-degree angle with your palms facing up. Do not place your hands above your shoulders. Leaving your left foot on the floor, cross your right ankle over the left knee.

Rotate your right ankle-on-knee to the left, so that your right foot touches the floor. Be sure not to move your left foot; it should only roll to accommodate the rotation. You do not want your left foot to move further away; that would decrease the effect of the exercise. Turn your head to the right. If it is comfortable, press your right knee toward your left foot, opening the hip more, but press only until you feel the stretch. Hold this position for 1 minute, then switch sides and repeat.

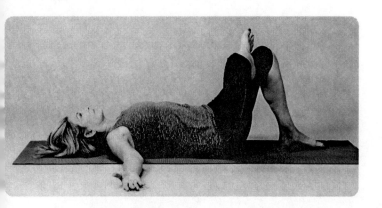

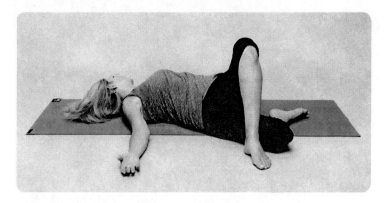

5. Standing Quad Stretch

Stand with your feet hip-width apart and parallel. Place one foot up on a chair seat behind you, while holding onto the back of another chair for balance. Be sure to keep your knees even and your hips level while your foot is on the chair. Hold for 1 minute, then carefully remove that foot from the chair, place your other foot onto the chair, and repeat the exercise.

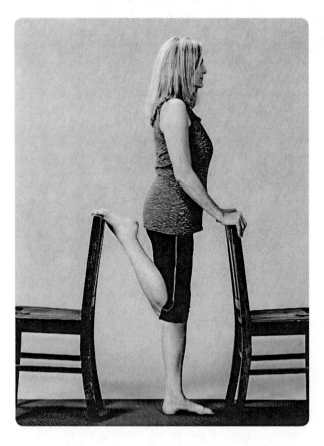

6. Cats and Dogs

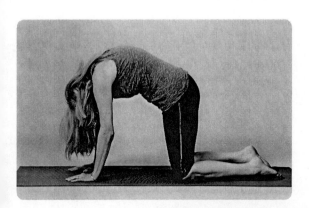

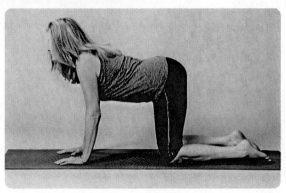

Move onto your hands and knees. Be sure that your hips are above your knees and your shoulders are above your wrists. Arch your back up, while tucking your head and hips down. Then arch your back down, while lifting your head and sticking your butt up. Breathe out when your back arches up, and breathe in when your back arches down. Move up and down 10 times.

Exercises to Prepare for Golf/Tennis

This routine is designed for the person who is feeling better but wants to maintain better posture, alignment, and function while playing tennis or golf. The demand of this routine is more than the demand for the previous exercises that focused on chronic pain. Ideally, if you are having back pain, you first should do the routine designed for your back pain or whichever routine that focuses on your pain. Once you are feeling better, you can move to this routine.

The best time to do this routine is before and after you play.

1. Sitting Arm Circles with Block

Sit on the edge of a chair. Place your feet hip-width apart. Roll your hips forward to create a small arch in your low back. Place a small block between your knees. You may substitute a small ball, but be sure it will keep your knees hip-width apart. Slightly squeeze the block at your knees. Extend your arms to the sides at shoulder height with your palms facing down, then move your arms back slightly. Pinch your shoulder blades back and down, while sticking out your chest. Rotate your arms forward in little, two-inch circles. Do 40 circles.

In the same position, turn your palms up, and rotate your arms in small circles backwards 40 times.

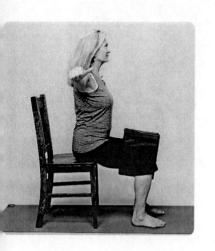
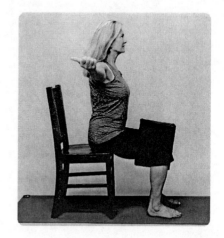

2. Sitting Elbow Touches with Block

Sit on the edge of a chair. Place your feet hip-width apart. Roll your hips forward to create a small arch in your low back. Place a small block between your knees and slightly squeeze it. With your hips rolled forward, place your knuckles on your temples with your thumbs pointing down. Touch your elbows together, keeping them level. Then pull your elbows open and back as far as you comfortably can. Repeat this exercise 30 times.

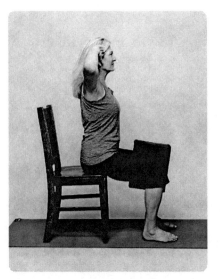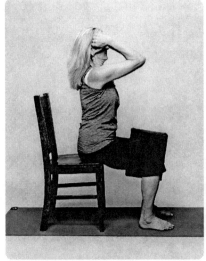

3. Assisted Runner Stretch

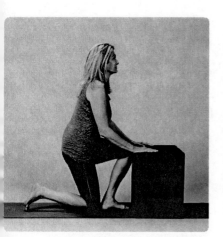 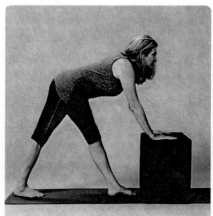

Kneel several inches in front of a chair or large block. Place the toes of your right foot at the edge of the chair (block). Place your left knee on the floor immediately behind the heel of your right foot. Curl your left foot up onto its toes.

Then stand up, while keeping your hands on the block. Try to get both feet flat on the floor. Straighten both legs and tighten your thigh muscles. With your hands still on the chair (block), roll your hips and stick your butt up. Try to arch your back down while rolling your hips. As you get better at this, you can bend your elbows, while keeping your legs straight and rolling your hips. Hold for 1 minute, then change sides and repeat the exercise.

4. Upper Spinal Floor Twist

Lie on your side in a fetal position with your arms together and straight out in front of you, and with your bent knees together at belly button height. Rotate your top arm and upper body to the other side. Place the hand of your bottom arm on your knees. Turn your head to follow the arm that is opening up. Be sure to keep your knees together while you are in this position. Breathe and relax your arm and shoulder. Let gravity do the work, and don't force the arm to the floor. Hold for 1 minute, then rotate your arm and body back to your initial fetal position. Roll to your other side and repeat the exercise.

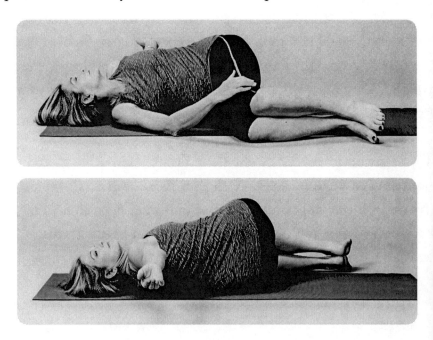

5. Back Extension on Elbows

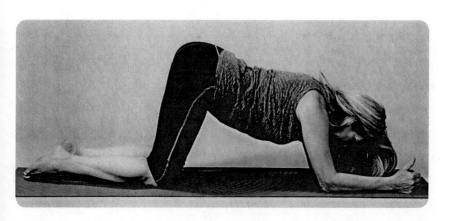

Start on your hands and knees, making sure your hips are directly above your knees and your wrists are directly below your shoulders. Move your hands one hand-length forward, then place your elbows on the floor where your hands were. This should move your hips slightly forward of your knees. Roll your hips to create an arch in your low back. Allow your shoulder blades to come together and your chest to fall towards the floor. Hold for 1 minute.

Exercises to Prepare for Walking/Running

As mentioned earlier, I believe walking is the best exercise for the body. Everyone should do it every day. The more you walk, the better you will feel. If you are having chronic pain and walking hurts, do the menu for your specific issue from the chronic pain section first. Once you are feeling better and can walk without pain, you should start walking.

This routine is a good postural bridge from the negative stimulus of everyday activities into better movement. Do this routine before and after you walk, and you will get more enjoyment from your walk.

If you are a runner, I recommend walking before your run. Take 10 minutes before each run and simply walk a bit. Then after you run, you should walk another 10 minutes. The body moves differently when you run. By walking before and after you run, you allow your body to warm up and cool down.

This routine will prepare your body for walking or running.

1. Cross Crawl

Lie on your back with your legs straight and your arms at your sides. Keeping your elbows straight, lift one arm over your head and touch the floor with your hand. At the same time lift the opposite knee to your chest. Keep the leg that remains on the floor straight. Move your arm and leg back to the floor, and then perform the same movement with the other arm and leg. Do 20 pairs of these.

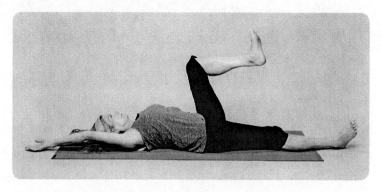

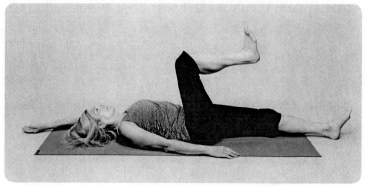

2. Hip Lift

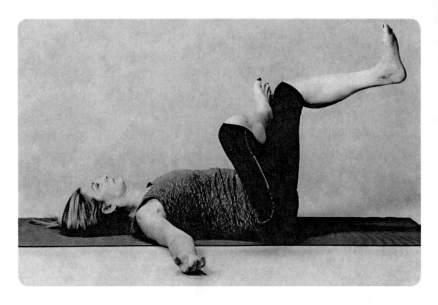

Lie on your back with your feet hip-width apart and your knees comfortably bent. Cross your right ankle over your left knee. Then lift your left knee to a 90-degree angle with the right ankle still in place. Flex your left foot back as you hold your left leg in the proper angle. Be sure to keep your left knee in line with the hip. Press your right knee toward your left foot as you try to hold the position. Hold for 1 minute, then change sides and repeat the exercise.

3. Sitting Floor Twist

Sit on the floor with your legs extended straight out. Cross your right foot to the outside of your extended left leg. Tighten your left thigh and flex your left foot back. Do not let your extended leg rotate out. Cross your left elbow over to your right knee, and twist your shoulders to the right. Try to roll your booth hips up and extend out your chest. Be sure to use your shoulders to twist and not pressing too hard with your elbow at your knee. Lightly prop yourself up with your right arm. Hold for 1 minute, then change sides and repeat.

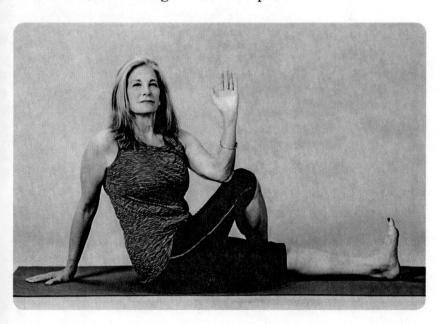

4. Cats and Dogs

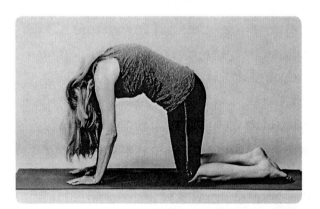

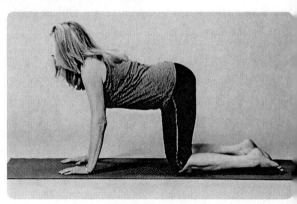

Move onto your hands and knees. Be sure that your hips are above your knees and your shoulders are above your wrists. Arch your back up, while tucking your head and hips down. Then arch your back down, while lifting your head and sticking your butt up. Breathe out when your back arches up, and breathe in when your back arches down. Move up and down 10 times.

5. Sitting Knee Pillow Squeezes

Sit on the edge of a chair. Place your feet hip-width apart, with your feet pointed straight ahead. Be sure they do not point out, and be sure they are in line with each other (with the outer sides of the feet parallel). There should be a 90-degree bend in your knees. Roll your hips forward to create a slight arch in your low back. Pull your shoulders back and down, sticking out your chest. Place a block between your knees. You may substitute a small ball for the block. Squeeze the block with your knees. Relax your ab muscles and remember to breathe. Squeeze the block 60 times, while maintaining the body position.

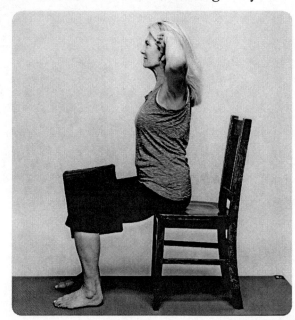

6. Counter Stretch

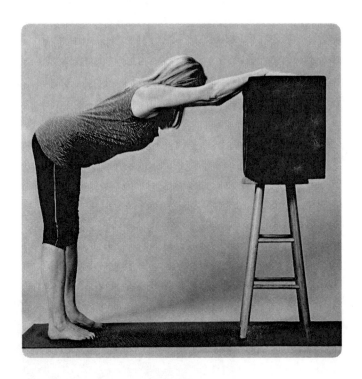

   While standing, place your hands on an elevated surface that is about chest height. Move your chest downward, extending your arms out straight. Adjust your feet so that they are directly below your hips, keeping them straight (parallel) and hip-width apart. Flex your thigh muscles, keeping the knees straight. Roll your hips, putting an arch in your low back and allowing your upper body to sink further down. Hold for 1 minute.

Final Words

The Pain-Free Life Program is a process of exercises that will start you on a journey of empowering yourself to feel better and stay active as you grow older. If you have pain, this book gives you the tools to be proactive toward achieving better muscle balance and better posture, which eliminates biomechanical dysfunction. This will ultimately create less pain and less breaking down of your body.

Regardless of your current activity and fitness level, this book will help you understand how to achieve proper motion and proper alignment. Don't ignore the need for motion. Don't ignore your body's signals. You must take responsibility and do what your body has been designed for 200,000 years to do. You must get back the natural design of the human body. That can only happen through better posture. As the saying goes, every journey begins with one step. This book is your first step to feeling better.

Don't delay, get up and move!

DO YOU WANT MORE?

Some readers will be able to use the exercises included in this book to feel better right away. Others will need to be more motivated. The results depend on you and your body, as well as how active you want to be and how limiting your pain is.

For those in need of more help and more direction than a book provides, I own Exercise Therapy of Kansas City, where we help clients on a one-on-one basis. You can also visit our website *www.exercisetherapykc.com* to see online courses and to schedule a personal consultation that can start you on your path of eliminating chronic pain and feeling better.

Community outreach is important to us and we are always looking for ways to reach more people with our message. Please contact us if you would like to arrange a speaking engagement for your business or organization.

About the Author

Travis Perret has been helping clients return to an active lifestyle without chronic pain for over 20 years. He has helped thousands of people move better and feel better through the Pain-Free Life Program.

Travis graduated from the University of Kansas and received his degree in Exercise Science with an emphasis in pre-physical therapy. He was a decathlete on the University of Kansas track and field team. After graduating, he moved to San Diego, California, to study the use of exercise and posture in helping those who have chronic pain. In 2004, he moved back to the Midwest and opened Exercise Therapy of Kansas City.

Travis lives in Overland Park, KS with his wife and two daughters. He loves spending time with his family and time in the outdoors.

You can follow Travis on his website:
www.exercisetherapykc.com

Or email him with
questions at *travis@exercisetherapykc.com*.

CPSIA information can be obtained
at www.ICGtesting.com
Printed in the USA
LVOW12s0315191117
556876LV00001B/2/P